Health In

(formerly Computers in Health Care)

Kathryn J. Hannah   Marion J. Ball
Series Editors

Springer
New York
Berlin
Heidelberg
Hong Kong
London
Milan
Paris
Tokyo

Health Informatics Series
(formerly Computers in Health Care)

(continued after Index)

Florian Leiner   Wilhelm Gaus
Reinhold Haux   Petra Knaup-Gregori

Medical Data Management
A Practical Guide

Foreword by Dr. Gustav Wagner

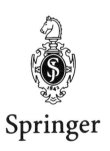

Springer

Florian Leiner, PhD
(Adjunct Lecturer at the University for
    Health Informatics and Technology
    Tyrol, Innsbruck, Austria)
Stuckstrasse 4
D-81677 Munich, Germany
FlorianLeiner@web.de

Wilhelm Gaus, PhD
Department of Biometry and
    Medical Documentation
University of Ulm
Schwabstrasse 13
D-89075 Ulm, Germany

Reinhold Haux, PhD
Institute for Health Information Systems
University for Health Informatics and
    Technology Tyrol
Innrain 98
A-6020 Innsbruck, Austria

Petra Knaup-Gregori, PhD
Institute of Medical Biometry and
    Informatics
University of Heidelberg
Im Neuenheimer Feld 400
D-69120 Heidelberg, Germany

Series Editors:

Kathryn J. Hannah, PhD, RN
Adjunct Professor, Department
    of Community Health Science
Faculty of Medicine
The University of Calgary
Calgary, Alberta, Canada

Marion J. Ball, Ed.D.
Vice President, Clinical Solutions
Healthlink
2 Hamill Road
Quadrangle 359 West
and
Adjunct Professor
The Johns Hopkins University
    School of Nursing
Baltimore, MD, USA

Cover art © 2002 by Roy Wiemann.

With 7 figures.

Library of Congress Cataloging-in-Publication Data
Medizinische Dokumentation. English.
    Medical data management / editors, Florian Leiner . . . [et al.].
        p. ; cm. — (Health informatics)
    A Practical Guide.
    Includes bibliographical references and index.
    ISBN 0-387-95159-8 (softcover)   ISBN 0-387-95594-1 (hardcover)   (alk. paper)
    1. Medical records—Data processing.   2. Database management.   3. Medicine—Data
processing.   4. Information storage and retrieval systems.   I. Leiner, F. (Florian)   I. Title.
III. Series.
    [DNLM: 1. Medical Records.   2. Forms and Records Control—methods.   3. Information
Storage and Retrieval.   4. Information Systems.   WX 173 M4879 2002a]
    R864.M476   2002
    651.5´04261—dc21   2002070549

ISBN 0-387-95159-8   (softcover)   ISBN 0-387-95594-1   (hardcover)   Printed on acid-free paper.

Authorized translation of the third German language edition Leiner F, Gaus W, Haux R. *Medizinische Dokumentation*
© 1999 by F.K. Schattauer Verlag GmbH, Stuttgart - New York.

Printed in the United States of America.

9 8 7 6 5 4 3 2 1   SPIN 10785042   (softcover)   SPIN 10894053   (hardcover)

Typesetting: Pages created by the authors using MS Word 97.

www.springer-ny.com

Springer-Verlag   New York Berlin Heidelberg
A member of BertelsmannSpringer Science+Business Media GmbH

To
Professor Herbert Immich
1917–2002

Foreword to the First German Edition

Modern medicine is characterized by the continuously growing spectrum of improving diagnostic methods and therapeutic processes. It keeps getting more complicated and confusing and therefore also needs more order.

The main goal of medical documentation is to provide information for the adequate care of patients. Carefully carried out written records like a patient history, physician indexes, or, more recently, patient databases serve to reach this goal.

Moreover, progress in clinical medicine is based on the exchange of experiences that are themselves largely based on the uniform entry, use, and analysis of comparable data and findings obtained from unhealthy participants. National and international institutions have been trying for years to come up with premises for this. The so-called "Blue Books" of the World Health Organization (WHO) for the standardization of the histological classification of tumors, the International Classification of Diseases for Oncology (ICD-O) for the standardized recording of tumor localization and morphology, and the TNM-System and TNM-Atlas of the International Union Against Cancer (UICC) for the documentation of studies of tumors are cited, for example, in the clinical oncology sector. The existence of classification systems has cleared the way for the modern, internationally accepted documentation of medically interesting matters.

The increased specifications in health structure law regarding the creation of physician reports as well as lawmakers' and the medical associations' increased efforts to improve quality assurance in medicine require the detailed documentation of patient-based data and findings. The fact that carefully designed medical documents are of value for physicians (e.g., for legal disputes) as well as for patients in critical situations where the documentation could be lifesaving is only briefly mentioned.

The fascination of the possibilities in medicine that have been made available through computers unfortunately relegated knowledge about the importance of careful documentation to the background in past years.

In 1975, the field was described in the *Handbook of Medical Documentation and Data Processing*. Today, 20 years later, there are many books that cover an aspect of the field. But a book about the core theme of medical informatics has not been written. It is therefore even more welcome that the authors of this textbook handle the theme in detail in consideration of new technological advances. They also prove the relevance of medical documentation as needed for optimal patient care and clinical research.

A requirement gap that has been around for a long time has finally been closed with this introduction on hand. Interested physicians and students of medicine, medical informatics, and informatics, such as medical documentors and documenting assistants, will greet the arrival of this textbook and find it useful.

Prof. Dr. Gustav Wagner
Heidelberg, Germany
June 1995

Series Preface

This series is directed to health care professionals who are leading the transformation of health care by using information and knowledge. Launched in 1988 as Computers in Health Care, the series offers a broad range of titles: some addressed to specific professions such as nursing, medicine, and health administration; others to special areas of practice such as trauma and radiology. Still other books in the series focus on interdisciplinary issues, such as the computer-based patient record, electronic health records, and networked health care systems.

Renamed Health Informatics in 1998 to reflect the rapid evolution in the discipline now known as health informatics, the series will continue to add titles that contribute to the evolution of the field. In the series, eminent experts, serving as editors or authors, offer their accounts of innovations in health informatics. Increasingly, these accounts go beyond hardware and software to address the role of information in influencing the transformation of health care delivery systems around the world. The series also will increasingly focus on "peopleware" and organizational, behavioral, and societal changes that accompany the diffusion of information technology in health services environments.

These changes will shape health services in the next millennium. By making full and creative use of the technology to tame data and to transform information, health informatics will foster the development of the knowledge age in health care. As coeditors, we pledge to support our professional colleagues and the series readers as they share advances in the emerging and exciting field of health informatics.

Kathryn J. Hannah
Marion J. Ball

Preface

Careful documentation is essential in all fields of medicine and health care, whether it may serve the treatment of patients, compliance with legal obligations, reimbursement and cost analysis, quality assurance, or clinical research. Clinical documentation must be conducted in a systematic way; otherwise, there is a danger of it becoming a tiresome affair, consuming an excessive amount of time and money, and being of hardly any use.
This book describes the basic concepts of clinical documentation and data management. We have tried to keep it as simple as possible—but not simpler.
The book is intended to assist you in designing and using clinical documentation and data management systems. We present the most relevant clinical coding systems (e.g., for coding diagnoses) and typical clinical documentation (e.g., the patient record). Hospital information systems and clinical studies are very important application areas of clinical documentation; we give an overview of both. Our thesaurus makes up a good part of the book. Use it to look up definitions and relations of the concepts treated in the book. All concepts defined in the thesaurus are set in **boldface** the first time they appear in a chapter.

Subject, goals, and contents of the book

The book is geared toward students who are trained in clinical documentation and data management, for example in the areas of medicine and medical/health informatics, as well as health information managers. As an introduction, it is also suitable for physicians, nurses, and other health care professionals who design or use clinical data management systems.

Who should read this book?

The authors offer the information contained in this book in the form of lectures mainly for students of medical/health informatics and health information management, but also for medical students and physicians. Depending on thoroughness and the background of the audience, the complete material can be taught in about 12 to 24 hours of instruction. The audience should command the most basic medical knowledge, particularly some medical terminology.
We recommend that instructors accompany the lectures with practical exercises of the use of clinical data management systems and clinical coding systems. Provide your students with real coding systems and—to cite just two examples—have them code diagnoses with the ICD and stage cases with the TNM system.

How to impart information?

Corresponding German edition

The first German edition of this book appeared in 1995. This English edition corresponds to the Third German edition of 1999.

Acknowledgments

In preparing this book, many persons supported us in various ways. We express our gratitude to all of them, even if we can name only a few here.

Invaluable advice came from our colleagues of the German Society of Medical Informatics, Biometry, and Epidemiology, particularly from the Working Group on Medical Documentation and Classification. Special thanks go to Birgit Brigl, Karl-Heinz Ellsässer, Ewald Glück, Stefan Gräber, Bernd Graubner, Rüdiger Klar, Tibor Kesztyüs, and Martin Schurer.

To translate a book into a foreign language and publish it with an international scope is an ambitious project. We would not have succeeded without the help and support of Anita Lagemann, Marion Ball, Frieda Kaiser, Merida Johns, and Jeremy Wyatt.

The authors have been greatly influenced by Herbert Immich, former director of the Institute of Medical Documentation, Statistics and Data Processing at the University of Heidelberg. We dedicate this book to him.

Not least, we want to thank our students who kept asking critical questions and drew our attention to incomplete and indistinct arguments.

Florian Leiner
Munich, Germany

Wilhelm Gaus
Ulm, Germany

Reinhold Haux
Innsbruck, Austria

Petra Knaup-Gregori
Heidelberg, Germany

March 2002

Contents

What Is Medical Documentation About? 1

Documentation denotes the methods and activities of collecting, **coding**, ordering, storing, and retrieving **information** to fulfill specific future tasks.

Information is often contained in **documents**. To retrieve documents containing a specific piece of information, they previously must have been **coded** correctly.

This **definition** clarifies it: Documentation is no end in itself. Information is only documented in order to use it later on—without this, collecting, labeling, ordering, and storing would be useless. Thus, documentation is meant to put information at the disposal of authorized persons in a purposeful manner. To be precise: it must be presented completely, without **noise**, at the right time, at the right place, and in the right form. Therefore, documentation can be said to serve **information and knowledge logistics**.

In this chapter you will learn

- the central significance of **medical documentation** for medicine, i.e., for **patient care** as well as for medical research;
- that medical documentation does not have to be taken as an unavoidable fate but that it is most important to set goals and to proceed systematically to achieve them with the least amount of effort;
- what objectives and results a documentation can attain;
- why methods for documentation have to be chosen carefully for the specific objectives; why these methods have to be applied with proficiency; and why good documentation is always a matter of both diligence and creativity;
- the potential of **computer-based data management systems**, and why the **computer** doesn't automatically make documentation better.

What It Is and What It Isn't 1.1

Medical documentation can deal with very different kinds of information. These reflect the different objectives and tasks of documentation that, on the other hand, require the use of different documentation methods.

Since we cannot completely cover the wide variety of objectives and methods, the main focus of this book is on the documentation of statements related to the illness and medical care of individual patients. This kind of documentation, which we **term clinical**

documentation, typically contains information about the history, the symptoms, clinical findings, diagnoses, therapies, and prognosis of a patient's illness.

This does not mean that we will ignore, for example, caregiving documentation, the documentation of medical textbook knowledge, or epidemiological databases completely. But we will deal with them only where they relate to our main focus.

What about nursing documentation?

In Germany, medical documentation stands for a **concept** that includes the contributions of all health care professions. So, in our definition and usage, **nursing documentation** is a specification, or sort, of medical documentation.

1.2   Medical Documentation: Do We Really Need It?

... since it's so boring

Medical documentation within the context of patient care sometimes seems to be just tedious form-filling or drudgery at the computer. Who really needs documentation? Does it serve only bureaucracy? Who takes advantage of it? Questions like these are discussed in the following section.

1.2.1   Problems and Motivation

Is it worthwhile?

A lot of documentation takes place in our hospitals and doctors' practices. A university hospital, for example, produces roughly 6 million documents (discharge summaries, laboratory results, etc.) per year. Storing these documents conventionally on paper would mean that about 1.5 kilometers of filing space are needed for **patient records**. What makes all this effort worthwhile?

First, appropriate **recording** of **data** is necessary for the accurate, continuous treatment of a patient. Records contain statements about the course of the treatment made by another person at an earlier place and time.

Certain data have to be acquired according to legal and other regulations. When going to court, it is important not only that a required action had been taken but also that it was documented.

Certainly, documentation is also done for administrative purposes: After all, it is important that expenses stay within reasonable bounds and that **health care interventions** are adequately reimbursed.

Measures taken to ensure the **quality of patient care** are, to a considerable extent, based on the documentation of treatment data. The same applies to clinical research activities, which play an important role, at least at university hospitals.

More Important Today Than Ever Before

Hippocrates recommended the **acquisition** of patient data to his students. However, there has been a growing impression in recent decades that traditional documentation methods are no longer sufficient. What led to this impression?

First of all, today's diagnostics are much more complex than ever before. Many diagnostic actions result in an immense amount of quantitative and qualitative findings that need to be assessed together.

Nowadays, extreme division of labor in patient care is common. This leads to a high demand for **communication** between all health professionals, laboratories, etc. Moreover, there is greater regional mobility among patients, and they are more prepared to change doctors from time to time.

Due to the successes of modern medicine, especially concerning acute diseases, the chronic diseases and multimorbidity at advanced ages play a more important role today. Therefore, clinical manifestations are getting more and more complex.

New documentation tasks, mainly for legal and financial purposes, have been added to the traditional ones. The use of computers enables extensive documentation and many diverse analyses. This fosters the wish to use the stored data on a large scale, e.g., for scientific research.

What Are the Objectives of Medical Documentation?

The motivation for medical documentation can be expressed in general terms, i.e., in an abstract way, as well as with reference to the concrete contents that should be documented. We will specify this in the following sections, restricting ourselves to clinical documentation (see above).

General Objectives

In the introduction of this chapter we already the general, abstract objective of medical documentation: to provide authorized persons with all relevant information (but not more) about one or several patients and their treatment, at the right time, at the right place, and in the right form.

Virtually every word of this phrase points to a whole range of requirements. "Authorized persons" requires taking complex access control structures into consideration; "all relevant information" requires mechanisms for ensuring the **completeness** of data and for the filtering of unnecessary detail or noise; "at the right time" puts great demands on the technical and organizational aspects of a system; "at the right place" is aimed at flexible and powerful concepts and tools for the transport of information; "in the right form" implies elaborate methods for processing and presenting information.

Based on this very general wording you cannot tell what the objectives of a concrete **data management system** are. Who are the authorized persons? What is the relevant information, and what should it be relevant for, anyway? We will deal with these questions in the next section. We would like to consider these general objectives as a sort of guideline for the formulation of complete and useful objectives of a data management system.

1.3.2 Objectives in Patient Care

Makes patient care more effective and appropriate

In the end, the most important objective of medical documentation is to contribute to effective and appropriate medical care for each individual patient. For each patient, the data management system has to provide all data that are relevant to decisions about diagnostic, therapeutic, or nursing interventions (i.e., health care interventions).

As a reminder, documentation helps to remember observations and health care interventions—be they finished, in progress, or still at a planning stage. As a communication aid, documentation supports the exchange of information between health care professionals. A patient record, for instance, fulfills both of these functions by bridging the time between two stays in a hospital, and by bridging the change of health professionals caring for the patient during these stays. Instead of exchanging patient records, communication between **health care institutions** usually occurs in the form of summary reports (e.g., discharge summaries, result reports, etc.).

There is another medical documentation task with a more limited scope in time and place: it supports the organization of health care interventions, for example, by recording test orders, treatment plans, and readmission dates.

1.3.3 Objectives in Administration

Forms the basis for refunding, process planning, and control

In the administrative sector, medical documentation can support a health care institution (for example, a hospital) in getting appropriate reimbursement for its services and in selecting and designing efficient work processes.

Since reimbursement depends to a great degree on the amount of services, there is a significant need for timely, reliable, and complete information about the performed interventions. The board of directors of a health care institution also has to plan and control the institution's work processes. Here, medical documentation helps to increase transparency by allocating the institution's costs to the providers and the receivers of services.

A number of implications arise for the appropriate documentation of patient care with regard to legislation and jurisdiction. In the event of legal proceedings, an inadequate amount of documentation can have negative implications for the health care institution. Liability claims can be expected when documentation systems aren't used correctly, or aren't used at all.

Depending on a country's regulations for reimbursement or accreditation, there are a number of obligations for an institution's documentation procedure.

Objectives in Quality Management and Education

1.3.4

Supports critical reflection and systematic monitoring

There is an ethical—and, in many countries, a legal—obligation for health care providers to ensure a high quality of patient care. The goal of medical documentation is to support the **quality management** of a health care institution, especially by providing appropriate information:
- in retrospect for the critical reflection on individual courses of illness (medical audit), and
- for systematic **quality monitoring** (where certain **attributes** of selected types of health care interventions are continually checked).

Medical documentation can be a valuable tool for the education and training of health care professionals. There are two primary functions:
- to provide a record for the critical evaluation of a student's actions and assessments, and
- to provide exemplary and realistic clinical problems and descriptions of courses of illness.

Objectives in Clinical Research

1.3.5

Allows patient selection and statistical analysis

The objective of clinical research is to generalize the experiences drawn from the care of individual patients, and to describe the rules that can be derived from those generalizations. Medical documentation can contribute to this objective as follows:

- by providing appropriate information for the critical evaluation of individual courses of illness in order to detect starting points for generalizations;
- by enabling the selection of patients with specific characteristics (e.g., all male patients with anterior myocardial infarction). This selection then forms the basis for a scientific study that has to be planned and documented separately;
- by providing particular data about a well-defined set of patients that enter into a planned evaluation study (for example, analyzing the frequency of stomach trouble after taking a pain-killer).

1.4   Multiple Use of Patient Data

Capture it once, use it extensively

Quite often, the same patient data are acquired several times for different objectives at different locations (not only patient data, but this is our main focus). In fact, the staff and patient expenses that arise from this cannot be justified. Computer-based data management systems offer the possibility of the **multiple use of data** recorded once to be used for different objectives and tasks.

A surgeon encodes, for example, a patient's diagnosis and therapy for the operation report. After the patient's discharge, this report forms the basis of the discharge report. The discharge report is the most important document for communication with the outpatient clinic or the practitioner taking over the care of the patient. Data on diagnosis and therapy are also important elements of problem lists, progress notes, nursing records, etc. They are necessary items for studies in quality management. In many countries, reimbursement depends in some way on diagnoses and therapies. Finally, the efficient management of a health care institution requires the treatment costs (e.g., consumption of material and drugs) to be contrasted with the kind and severity of the patient's illness, characterized by diagnosis and therapy.

Problems

Fig. 1.1 is a diagram of the basic problem regarding the multiple use of data: Depending on the question you pose and your viewpoint, your information need will be different. For the treatment of a patient, you will need a complete and concise overview of all data that are relevant for the decisions in that particular case; for a scientific study, comparability and **reliability** are of primary interest, which means that there will be a well-defined selection of (possibly very few) attributes of all patients of the **study sample**.

It has to be planned

The multiple use of patient data can actually only be ensured when the following conditions are met:

- All tasks of the data management system and all questions for analysis have been arranged beforehand.
- The demands on the quality of the data depend on the most ambitious task. (For example, the result of a physical examination may be formulated in free terms for the purpose of individual patient care. For a **clinical study**, on the other hand, some attributes have to be **captured** completely and follow clear guidelines, whereas other attributes do not have to be taken into account at all.)

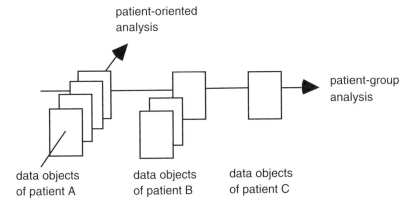

Fig. 1.1   Diagram of the multiple use of patient data: patient-oriented versus patient-group analyses as an example to demonstrate different information needs for different objectives of documentation.

When patient data within a certain field shall be used in multiple ways, documentation has to be planned and coordinated between all persons involved in order to fulfill the above-mentioned conditions.

The use of data for a task that has not been taken into account during the planning of the data management system can pose great problems. Technically it can be facilitated by **standardized documentation**, but this will not guarantee the data's semantical suitability for the new task.

Medical Documentation: Child's Play?   1.5

The most annoying part of documentation is that it often seems to take an unreasonable amount of time. This is particularly true when documentation is carried out unskillfully—not to say amateurishly. Selecting incorrect documentation methods (or using correct methods in the wrong way) produces a lot of unnecessary work, and often even leads to incorrect conclusions being drawn from the documentation.

Do it right —or leave it

Unnecessary expenses often arise when the same data are acquired repeatedly for different tasks instead of using the information in multiple ways (see section 1.4).

On the other hand, each analysis goal makes certain demands on the documentation's quality, e.g., with respect to its completeness of attributes and of **data objects**, its accuracy in every detail, and its conformity. Analyzing data without having selected appropriate documentation methods right from the start entails the risk of substantial misinterpretations. The research funds spent in that way could have been used elsewhere much more efficiently!

1.6   Computer-Supported Medical Documentation: A Panacea?

Computers support good and bad concepts

It is well known that computers aid in documentation. But this is only true when, in the course of introducing computer support, the documentation's structure has been reviewed critically. Otherwise, it is to be expected that bad documentation will be faithfully transformed into bad computer-based documentation. From a technical point of view, a computer tremendously extends the possibilities of storing and analyzing data. This fact creates the temptation to record "everything" in the vain hope of possessing the answers to all possible questions. There are three points we want to make about computer-based medical documentation:

- The basic methodology for documentation is to a great extent independent of the **storage medium**.
- The use of computers requires additional methods, for example for the construction of **computer-based application systems**, for database design, or for computer-based communication.
- The use of computers can have great advantages over conventional documentation (e.g., the simultaneous availability of data at different places, fast and secure data processing, a decrease in work load) but can have disadvantages as well (e.g., more awkward use or higher expenses). Through the use of a computer, documentation often gets more abstracted and quite often inscrutable, so that incorrect data or mistakes in operating the program go unnoticed in many cases (black-box effect).

1.7   Checklist: Objectives of Medical Documentation

Checklist

The general objective of information and knowledge logistics in medicine is:

To make available the right medical information (e.g., about a patient) and the right **medical knowledge** (e.g., about a disease) at the right time, at the right place, to the right persons, in the right form.

Specific objectives of concrete data management systems typically are:
- to support patient care (to remind staff of and communicate information, to help in organizing the care process);
- to fulfill external obligations (legal requirements, accreditation, and reimbursement regulations);
- to support administration (in planning, controlling, and re-funding the health care institution's services);
- to support quality management (by enabling critical reflection and systematic monitoring of processes);
- to support scientific research (by enabling patient selection and **statistical analysis**);
- to support clinical education (by providing information for critical review and case examples).

Generally, each piece of information within a **medical data management system** can serve many of these objectives, provided the system has been planned carefully.

Exercises

1.8

Exercise 1

Give some reasons why medical documentation became more significant in recent decades.

Exercise 2

What are the general objectives of medical documentation?

Exercise 3

We stated: "Documentation is no end in itself." Give an example of documentation in your job or in your private life. Describe how you use this documentation.

Exercise 4

What do we mean by information logistics, and what is knowledge logistics? Give examples from your personal life.

Exercise 5

What is meant by multiple usability of patient data? Give reasons why the multiple usability of data is especially important in the field of health care. We mentioned some specific objectives for medical documentation in section 1.3. For which of them do you need to know
- that patient Adams has a penicillin allergy?
- that patient Evans suffered a wound infection after an operation?

Basic Concepts of Clinical Data Management and Coding Systems

The field of **medical documentation** maintains—like all **informa-tion** processing—a remote (and often clumsy) technical language. But even the most impressive specialist **terms** vary in usage and understanding depending on the person. Therefore, we want to introduce the basic **concepts** of medical documentation and ex-plain our technical language in this chapter. In addition, we have provided a **thesaurus** of medical documentation in Chapter 11, including an alphabetical list of the most important terms in the field together with their explanation (thesaurus entries are set in boldface in the text).

Introduction

Unfortunately, it may not be a particular pleasure for you to work through this chapter, although we tried to make it a bit easier with a lot of examples. You won't discover a great deal of linguistic beauty in our specialist terms. Nevertheless, we hope that you will gain from the conceptual clarity we strive for.

The Documenting Institution

2.1

Where and for whom is **documentation** carried out? To answer these questions we will introduce the most prevalent facilities for **patient care**. For each of these facilities, we will name the most important "stakeholders," or groups of persons whose information needs have to be met by a **data management system**.

Introduction

In this chapter you will learn
- the basic structure of the most important patient care facilities taking advantage of medical documentation;
- which professional groups in these institutions may have in-formation needs and must be considered when designing data management systems.

What will you learn?

The Physician's Office and the Outpatient Clinic

2.1.1

The most important working areas in a physician's office or in an outpatient clinic are the *examination and treatment rooms*.

Working areas

Moreover, there is an *administration area* for
- admission,
- billing,
- documentation,
- typing service, and
- telephone service.

Depending on specialty and equipment, a physician's office may have additional *functional areas*
- for diagnostics, e.g., x-ray or laboratory services, and
- for therapy, e.g., outpatient operating rooms or a physiotherapy department.

As an area of (involuntary) interest especially to patients, you shouldn't forget the *waiting area* with waiting rooms, rest rooms, etc.

Professional groups

The individual groups of persons in a physician's practice have different information needs.
Aside from the patient as a person who has a fundamental information need in every health care situation, there are essentially three groups in the physician's office or in the outpatient clinic:
- the physician(s),
- other health care professionals (e.g., nurses, laboratory staff, psychologists, physiotherapists)
- administrative staff.

The information needs of physicians in their offices are very comprehensive. For the other staff, they are somewhat more limited but shouldn't be underestimated. Think about the information needs of the receptionist answering the office telephone!

2.1.2   The Hospital

Working areas

The individual areas of a hospital can be characterized by their tasks. First of all, there are
- *inpatient areas* (with their wards and care facilities) and
- *outpatient departments* (including policlinics and emergency clinics).

Furthermore, in every hospital there are functional areas, or service units,
- for diagnostics (e.g., clinical chemistry, immunology, radiology),
- for therapy (e.g., operating rooms, physiotherapy, social therapy),
- and for ancillary functions (e.g., pharmacy, blood bank, medical records archives, hospital library, typing services for medical **documents**, computing services).

The *hospital administration* is composed of areas for
- central administration (e.g., staff administration, resource management, financial management),
- patient data management, billing, and reporting, and
- facility management, maintenance, supply, and waste disposal.

Finally, the *management areas* of a hospital and their particular information needs have to be considered, i.e., the administrative, medical, and nursing directors and their personal staff.

The individual professional groups in a hospital have different information needs. Essentially, these groups are

Professional groups

- physicians;
- nursing care professionals;
- administrative professionals;
- other health care professionals, providing diagnostic and therapeutic services;
- professionals in the field of medical informatics and documentation (including staff in the record archives).

Information needs can vary to a great degree even within a professional group. The information needs of ward physicians, laboratory doctors, and senior consultants differ.

Other Relevant Institutions

2.1.3

Apart from the institutions for primary patient care, several other institutions play important parts in the health care arena. Their specific roles and interests depend substantially on the organization of a country's health care system.

There is one generic function—to protect a person from the risk of unaffordable health care costs in the case of disease or injury—for which in virtually all countries there are health insurance organizations. They charge their clientele regular fees and "buy" medical

Health insurance organizations

services from health care providers for clients who are ill. Internationally, there are a multitude of political and organizational variations that are all derived from two prototypical forms: public and private health care insurance.

Public insurance

Public health care insurance is based on the principle of solidarity: members of a population pay a fee, or contribution, according to their financial abilities, and are entitled to an equal amount of health care services in case of illness. In its most general form, public insurance is a tax-paid public health system with state-employed providers (like in the United Kingdom, for example). A country's health system may commit certain members of the population (e.g., those with a lower income) to choose one out of a number of not-for-profit insurance organizations and pay contributions according to their income. In case of illness, the organizations pay for a common and state-regulated set of health care services; this is the situation in Germany, for example.

Private insurance

Private health care insurance is based on the principle of individual risk: the fee, or premium, that individuals pay (if they are healthy enough to be accepted as clients) depends on their individual risk of becoming ill, and is independent of their financial abilities. The premium further depends on the amount of health care services that have been arranged in the contract in case of an illness.

Health maintenance organizations

Health maintenance organizations (HMOs) constitute a specific form of private health insurance that don't buy single health care services for their clients but pay the providers a fixed sum, or capitation, for every person in their area of responsibility, regardless of the services provided. Capitation is meant to restrict the provision of medical services to those services indisputably necessary to restore or protect a healthy condition. Typically, capitation is supported by measures of *managed care*, further reducing unnecessary (or uncovered) services and securing minimal standards for the quality of care.

Information needs for insurance

The clinical information needs of every insurance system are chiefly characterized by two questions: Has the health care provider taken every measure necessary to restore the patient to a healthy (and cost-free) condition as well as to prevent the (expensive) deterioration of this condition in the future? And have any measures been taken that are not justified by these criteria, for which payment might be consequently refused?

Other organizations

In every country, there are a number of additional health care organizations like national or regional health care authorities, professional bodies, patient organizations, etc. To build and implement useful and accepted clinical data management systems, you should be familiar with the organizations that pertain to the field of application. Think twice about those organizations' interests and the possible contributions they can make before you start your project; it might pay in the long run.

From Attributes to Data Management

2.2

Introduction

In this chapter we introduce basic **terminology** and explain the concepts necessary for talking about medical documentation. The choice of concepts as well as the **definitions** we give reflect our experience and judgment. We follow generally approved definitions issued by the International Organization for Standardization (ISO).

In this chapter you will learn
- to apply the basic terminology of medical documentation,
- alternative terms and related concepts.

What will you learn?

Objects and Attributes

2.2.1

Definitions

An **object** represents a part of the perceptible or conceivable world (ISO standard no. 1087). Each single object exhibits a set of characteristics that may distinguish it from other objects or that display commonalities between the objects.

By determining common characteristics, a set of similar objects may be embraced by an abstract unit of thought called a concept, or an **object class**.

Within documentation, only selected object characteristics are represented in the form of **attributes**: For instance, one of the attributes **recorded** for an object might be "color of the surface: green." The first part of the expression is called the **attribute type**, the expression behind the colon is the **attribute value**. All possible values for an attribute type can be stated in advance in a **value set** (e.g., the set {red, blue, green, yellow} for the attribute type "color of the surface").

Objects can be of material or immaterial nature. The (fictitious) patient Angus Adams (date of birth: July 16, 1963), the (fictitious) **Ploetzberg Medical Center and Medical School** (PMC), and the (unfortunately real) disease tuberculosis are examples of objects. All these objects have a number of characteristics. Patient Adams weighs 68 kilograms and suffers from diabetes; the PMC has about 5000 employees and about 1500 beds; tuberculosis is caused by a mycobacterium.

Description and examples

More or less intuitively, we already assigned certain concepts to the objects in the examples above (we "typed" them): Mister Adams is a *patient*, Ploetzberg is a *hospital*, and tuberculosis is a *disease*.

Usually, you want to distinguish the objects belonging to a certain type and describe them in more detail. Thus, the concept is extended by a set of attribute types referring to the features of interest (but not to all, which would be impossible). To distinguish patients, one may chose, for example, the attribute types *surname*, *maiden name*, *first name*, and *date of birth*; for a detailed description one may choose the attribute types *weight in kilograms* and *diagnosis*. The value set for the weight might be the set of natural numbers; the value set for the diagnosis might be the set of **classes** of a disease **classification**.

So, within the documentation, an object is described only by the attribute values of the chosen attribute types (in short, by its attributes). In technical terms, the object is "represented" in the documentation by its attributes. A query of the documentation in the above example would yield only the name, date of birth, weight, and disease classes for any one patient.

Related concepts

"Is patient X already in the **computer**?" Surely, you have already heard statements like this, and maybe you hesitated for a moment and wondered who or what actually is in the computer. Basically, we have already given the answer to this question earlier; anyway, we want to make this important point very clear and take it a bit further.

First, we have to distinguish between the world outside the data management system and its—admittedly very restricted—image within the data management system (see Fig. 2.1). Certain concepts, or object classes, of the outside world may be chosen to be represented within documentation, e.g., patients, wards, **patient records**, or surgical operations.

But what is actually in the computer? In practical terms, it is the so-called **data objects**, or just **data**, which are stored, e.g., the character strings *Adams, Angus, 19630716,* and *m*. Of course, one has to agree at the outset on the meaning of, for example, *m* and *19630716*. It is only such agreements that make the data constitute information! Usually, the agreements take the form of **data object classes** which state, for example, that for each object of the object class "patient" the following data objects are to be recorded: surname, maiden name, first name, date of birth (in the format YYYYMMDD), and gender (*m* for male and *f* for female).

Thus, data objects are nothing but stored attribute values representing a certain **outside-world object** within the data management system. In contrast, data object classes are agreements on the attribute types and value sets that will be used for recording features of an outside-world object.

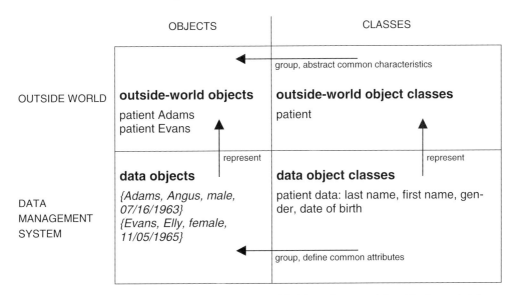

Fig. 2.1   Outside-world objects and outside-world object classes, data objects, and data object classes.
Outside-world objects and object classes are entities of the observed part of reality outside the data management system. Within the management system, they are represented by *data* objects and *data* object classes, respectively. Object *classes* are imaginary sets of objects, defined by their common characteristics (or attributes)—be it inside or outside the data management system.

Definitions, Labels, and Terminology

A definition is a statement that describes a concept and allows its differentiation from other concepts, using linguistic or other (e.g., formal) means.

A **label** is the representation of a concept, or of an object, using language, symbols, gestures, or other means. A purely linguistic label of a concept is called a term. Objects are often labeled with *names*.

Terminology is the entire stock of concepts (represented by their definitions) and labels in a specific subject field; it is also called a "specialist vocabulary." *Terminological knowledge* thus refers to the knowledge of a field's concepts, their meaning (i.e., their definitions), and their appropriate labels.

2.2.2

Definitions

Description and examples

As we explained in the last paragraph, a concept is a mental construct bringing together similar real-world objects, e.g., all disease states characterized by an inflammation of the stomach mucosa. The common label, or term, for this concept is "gastritis."

The terminology of a field can be made explicit in a systematic collection of its **specific concepts**. Typically, the entries of such collections are the specialist terms of the concepts in alphabetical order, followed by their definitions.
Everybody knows definitions from specialist dictionaries. The difficult thing with definitions is to explain the concept clearly, completely, and to avoid inconsistencies with other concepts in the terminology, using only terms that are either commonly known or explained elsewhere.

Related concepts

- **Synonyms** are different terms for the same concept.
  Example: *Whooping cough – Pertussis*
- Two **antonymous concepts** form a pair of opposites regarding at least one aspect while coinciding in the other aspects. They are both specializations of a common (generic) concept.
  Examples: *tachycardia – bradycardia* (with "abnormal heart rate" being the common concept),
  fever – hypothermia (but also: fever – normal temperature).
- A term is homony**mous** if it labels two or more different concepts.
  Examples: *lobe* as a synonymous term for "lung lobe" and for "brain lobe."
  SLE as an abbreviation for "systemic lupus erythematosus" or for "St. Louis encephalitis."
- A **generic concept** is the superordinate concept of a generic **concept relation**. It comprises the meaning of several subordinate concepts, called specific concepts.
  Example: Generic concept *Lung diseases;* Specific concepts *Pneumonia, Pulmonary emphysema, Pneumonedema.*
- **Intersecting concepts** share important characteristics, but differ in one or more aspects. Typically, they are specializations of a common (generic) concept.
  Example: *Toxic hepatitis – liver cirrhosis.*
- *Eponyms* are labels of concepts (in the medical field often diagnoses and therapeutic procedures) that contain the name of the person who has discovered or invented the concept.
  Examples: *Parkinson disease* (after James Parkinson, 1755–1824),
  Non-Hodgkin lymphoma (after Thomas Hodgkin, 1798–1866).

Data, Information, and Knowledge

Information is the knowledge about concrete objects, facts, or processes, which has a particular meaning within a certain context (e.g., in the context of health care)

Data constitute a formal and reinterpretable representation of information, suitable for **communication**, interpretation, and processing. Formalization may take the form of discrete characters or of continuous signals (e.g., sound signals). To be "reinterpretable," there has to be agreement on how data represent information.

Medical knowledge is information about the state of the art in the medical and health care domain at a given time with regard to terminology, established relations, and action guidelines. Thus, medical knowledge is medical information in a broader sense.

In the following, we will use the concept *information* in a narrower sense, i.e., as information about a patient and his or her medical care (e.g., information on Elly Evans, her medical history and her reaction to the beta-blocker administered during her last visit). The concept *medical knowledge* in this book stands for knowledge about diseases and clinical methods (e.g., knowledge about malaria or about digital subtraction angiography).

All documentation contains data. The crucial point of our definition is that data represent information, i.e., knowledge about concrete objects, facts, and processes. Looking back at the definitions of the previous section, this means the following: An attribute value within documentation represents information only if it is clear to which attribute type it belongs and which outside-world object it describes. A data item thus consists of at least the attribute type-value pair and a reference to the object it belongs to.

The attribute value "120" is meaningless without its attribute type "systolic blood pressure in mm Hg" and without the reference to the object "patient Angus Adams." Strictly speaking, it is still meaningless until you know that the measurement had been taken on April 4, 2001, at 2:30 P.M., after the patient had been lying recumbent for 10 minutes.

To ensure the correct assignment of data objects to outside-world objects and the correct interpretation of the attributes, the above-mentioned agreements are necessary. For that purpose, an unambiguous identification number might be added to all data objects (e.g., a patient number or a visit number), and the attribute types and their value sets might be cataloged (e.g., the range of tests offered by the laboratory as the value set for the attribute type "laboratory test").

Related concepts

Messages consist of data that are put together for transmission and are considered an entity for this purpose. The definition of "data" leads to the conclusion that the sender and receiver of a message have to agree about the identification of data objects and about the interpretation of attributes. Otherwise, the message could be misunderstood or even be incomprehensible.

A very important part of the agreements has to do with the value sets for the particular attribute types. The structure of the value set is crucial for the potential for use of that attribute, e.g., in **statistical analyses**. Different structures can be described on the basis of their **levels of measurement** (see Table 2.1). Two additional remarks concerning levels of measurement:
- Value sets of **qualitative attribute** types are based on classifications (see section 2.4.3)
- Values on an ordinal scale can be expressed by the elements of a numerical sequence (so-called ranks) in order to offer (restricted) possibilities for quantitative analyses.

Table 2.1. Levels of measurement that can be exhibited by the values of an attribute.

Attributes at a **quantitative level**: measurable or countable features. There are:
- **Ratio scale**: measurement variable with a true zero point; ratios of two measurements or frequencies can be computed and interpreted.
  Examples: body weight in kg, blood pressure in mm Hg, thrombozyte count.
  Ratio scales are always interval scales as well.
- **Interval scale**: measurement variable with a defined distance between any two values, but without a true zero point. Differences, but not ratios, can be computed and interpreted.
  Examples: body temperature, the calendar date.
  Taking the information loss, interval scales can always be reduced to an ordinal scale by a procedure called "ranking."

Attributes at a **qualitative level**: possible values form a set of labeled categories. There are:
- **Ordinal scale**: the categories have a meaningful order, or ranking. The observations can be sorted according to this order. In contrast to the interval scale, the differences between two attribute values are undefined.
  Example: stages of a disease, e.g., light, moderate, severe, very severe.
  Taking the information loss, ordinal scales can always be treated as a nominal scale.
- **Nominal scale**: the categories have names (Latin: nomina) and therefore no meaningful order, nor defined differences.
  Examples: gender, blood group.

Documents

2.2.4

Definitions

A document is a (more or less) structured accumulation of data, primarily intended for human perception. A document's data originate from (and reflect) a specific organizational context (e.g., an admission form is the record of an admission interview, a laboratory result sheet contains the results of one or more tests performed in the laboratory). The document can be exchanged as a unit between the users of a data management system or also between **application systems**.

The data objects contained in the document usually refer to a particular outside-world object—frequently the patient in **clinical documentation**.

A **document carrier** is any medium for the physical expression of a document. Document carriers may be sheets of paper, x-ray films, file cards (or other conventional media), but also magnetic disks, chip cards, optical disks (or other electronic media).

Description
and examples

Clinical documentation is traditionally characterized by the use of a multitude of documents, usually assigned to a certain patient. Examples of documents are admission forms, history sheets, laboratory requests, laboratory result reports, temperature curves, operation reports, anesthesia protocols, consultation reports, discharge summaries, etc. Paper is by far the most frequent document carrier, even if an increasing number of documents are stored—often redundantly—on a computer's magnetic disk.

There are typical structures for most of the common documents, recognizable almost all over the world. Nevertheless, the individual documents vary in structure to a considerable degree, even within a single institution. Intuitively, you might form a class of strongly structured documents (e.g., admission form, laboratory request, anaesthesia protocol) and a class of weakly structured documents (e.g., operation report, discharge summary). Variations in the first class naturally are smaller than in the second.

Data Management Systems

2.2.5

Definitions

A data management system accomplishes documentation tasks through
- organizational rules,
- conventional tools and aids, and
- application software installed on computers.

A data management system can store data in one way or another and usually is able to exchange messages with other systems.

Description and examples

The data management system of the department for pediatric surgery of the Ploetzberg Medical Center and Medical School consists of (paper-based) patient records; a computer network with application software supporting the composition of discharge summaries as well as the management of the patient records archive; and an index-card box with alphabetically sorted index-cards, used to refer to scientifically interesting cases. Explicitly or implicitly accepted organizational rules, concerning the record keeping, writing discharge summaries, filling in index-cards, etc., also form part of the data management system.

Which tools and rules are considered part of a certain data management system is determined pragmatically, in consideration of organizational, spatial, and staff point of views. The exchange of information and knowledge beyond the borders of the data management system may take the form of printed documents, electronic messages, or oral communication.

We do not consider the common patient database of the Ploetzberg Medical School to be part of the data management system of the pediatric surgery department, even if the department's patient data are entered into and retrieved from this database. The reason is that organizationally the central database is under the responsibility of hospital management and all departments have access to it. The database, however, exchanges electronic messages with the pediatric surgery's data management system, e.g., to inform it about new patient visits.

2.2.6   Exercises

Exercise 1

Object, concept, label, term, attribute type, and attribute value: Define these concepts in your own words. How are they related? Give examples.

Exercise 2

Hepatitis and jaundice: How are these two concepts related?

Exercise 3

Data, information, message, and knowledge: Define these concepts in your own words. How are they related? Give examples.

Exercise 4

Which level of measurement exhibits the values of the attribute "body temperature in degrees Fahrenheit"?

Exercise 5

In this chapter as well as in later ones we discuss hospitals. Give a few (perhaps five) attribute types that describe important aspects of the concept *hospital*. Given the values of these attributes, it should be possible to identify a hospital unambiguously and to make statements about its size and its diagnostic and therapeutic spectrum. Specify value sets for all attributes.

Document, data object, document carrier, and data management system: Define these concepts in your own words. How are they related? Give examples.

Exercise 6

Clinical Data Management Systems

2.3

Before we start to **classify** and describe the characteristics of data management systems in health care, we want to point out that in this chapter we do not restrict ourselves to clinical documentation—as in the rest of this book—but describe the whole range of medical documentation.

Introduction

In this chapter you will learn
- the most important aspects for analyzing and describing data management systems in health care, and
- how to use them.

What will you learn?

Characteristics of Clinical Data Management Systems

2.3.1

Because of the multitude of potential objectives of medical documentation, different objectives—and thus the different nature of the tasks—require different kinds of data management systems. In this section, we will discuss criteria that can be used to identify essential differences and similarities of individual data management systems. Such criteria will be very useful for the selection, construction, and evaluation of data management systems.
For every differentiating criterion, we will give a value set, or a number of choices, so that for any data management system exactly one of the choices is true (even if the decision will be difficult in some cases).

Characteristics

Distinction by Contents

2.3.1.1

The content of all medical documentation comes from three areas:

Clinical information is generally based on patient-related data. It describes characteristics of the patient, of the illness, and of the health care process. Clinical information can be found, for example, in patient records, or in the records of a therapeutic study. Clinical information in this sense is often called clinical facts or clinical results.

Clinical informa-tion ...

...vs. medical knowledge ...

Medical knowledge abstracts from the individual patient and describes general insights, e.g., about a certain disease (etiology, diagnostics, therapy, course, prognosis), or a certain diagnostic or therapeutic procedure (indication, execution, effectiveness, risks, etc.).

...vs. data on the health care system

Characteristics of the health care system basically provide statistical information about a health care system's infrastructure, often in a selected area (e.g., the distribution and availability of certain types of **health care institutions**, their average utilization rates, costs, etc.). Epidemiological data, e.g., the **incidence** of myocardial infarction of men between the ages of 50 and 60, may be considered part of the characteristics of a health care system as well as part of medical knowledge.

Classes

Let us say that a data management system belongs to exactly one of the following classes:

Class C1:   Contains primarily clinical information (clinical facts)

Class C2:   Contains primarily medical knowledge

Class C3:   Contains primarily characteristics of the health care system

Class C4:   Contains a balanced mixture of more than one of these information types

Class C9:   Cannot be assigned to one of the above

Example

The neurological outpatient clinic of the Ploetzberg Medical Center (PMC) runs a data management system that stores the clinical findings of patients. As an additional feature, the system provides context-sensitive access to selected neurological knowledge. Since the system's main emphasis lies on the **clinical findings documentation**, however, we will assign it to class C1.

As a precaution, we have added the residual class C9 in case it's impossible to assign a system to any of the other classes (e.g., because of missing information about the system).

2.3.1.2   Distinction by Utilization: Patient-Oriented or Grouped

Patient-oriented vs. grouped analysis

Analyzing medical documentation can be done with regard to one patient or to a group of patients. When choosing a therapy for one patient, for example, his or her specific diagnosis is of interest. The same diagnosis may, on the other hand, enter a calculation of diagnosis frequencies without reference to the patient (e.g., for an epidemiological study or for cost calculations). Thus, we distinguish patient-oriented (also case-based, or *casuistic)* and **patient-**

group analyses. **Patient-oriented analysis** is possible only if all attributes of interest refer to an identifiable patient. For that purpose, identifying attributes are recorded for every patient, usually the name, date of birth, and address.

The distinction between patient-oriented and patient-group analyses is of practical relevance: The focus of patient-oriented analyses is on the unambiguous identification of a patient and the adequate presentation of his or her data. A patient-group analysis produces statistical data such as frequencies or means. Here, the focus lies on comparability and on the correct interpretation of results.

Let us say that a data management system belongs to exactly one of the following classes:

Class U1: Aimed primarily at patient-oriented analysis
Class U2: Aimed primarily at patient-group analysis
Class U3: Aimed equally at patient-oriented as well as patient-group analyses
Class U9: Cannot be assigned to one of the above

Classes

Usually, both kinds of analyses are necessary, which is sensible since it wouldn't be economical to use two different data management systems with redundant data. Thus, the choice of the appropriate class and, more importantly, the choice of appropriate documentation methods, depends on the proportions of the two kinds of analyses in the mixture.

The data management system of PMC's neurological outpatient clinic supplies the health care process with the patients' data: this is a patient-oriented analysis. For the neurologist, however, it is just as important to analyze the database to gain additional knowledge, e.g., about prognostic factors of a certain disease: this is a patient-group analysis. Our conclusion: Class U3.

Example

Distinction by Level of Standardization

2.3.1.3

For documentation to be called standardized for a department, the data objects' attributes have to be *uniformly recorded* within that department.

What is being standardized?

For this purpose, it must be decided (1) which attribute types will be recorded, (2) using which possible values, and (3) for which data object classes. One might, for example, want to record the nutritional status, using the value set {cachetic, thin, normal weight, overweight, adipose, others}, of all inpatients during their admission examination.

**Added compa-
rability...**

Through standardization, *comparability* of data objects is achieved on two levels: On a formal level, it is ensured that the attributes needed for the comparison are recorded in identical terms for every object of interest. On a content level, the value set of an attribute type may provide a context that reduces the variability of meaning. In the example above, the term "thin" becomes far more precise by its being located between "cachectic" (the left extreme of the ordered set) and "normal weight" (its center) (cf. section 2.2.3, levels of measurement).

**... reduced
specificity**

The outcome of standardization is that many details of the actual situation are lost. In **standardized documentation** it usually isn't possible to depict a particular case in all its detail and distinctive features (as it is possible in **nonstandardized documentation** by formulating free text).

Classes

Let us say that a data management system belongs to exactly one of the following classes:
Class S1: Not standardized
Class S2: Partly standardized
Class S3: Mainly standardized
Class S4: Fully standardized
Class S9: Cannot be assigned to one of the above

The "edge" classes S1 and S4 are the exception: Almost all medical documentation contains standardized elements (even if it is only the calendar date or the case number). On the other hand, in patient care there is almost always a need to record the pecularities of a case in nonstandardized form (usually by using free text, see also terminology).

Example

The data management system of PMC's neurological outpatient clinic provides enumerative value sets for most of its attribute types (for numerical measures, a lower and upper bound are given together with the unit of measurement). Occasionally, free text is **allocated**, e.g., for the epicritical assessment of a case. We therefore decide on class S3.

2.3.1.4   **Distinction by Depth: Horizontal or Vertical Documentation**

The trade-off

The reliable operation of a clinical data management system with a given capacity always requires a trade-off: The more details have to be recorded for patient or case, the fewer patients or cases can be included in the documentation. Or the other way round: The more patients documented, the fewer details can be recorded.

So there is a fundamental limitation to the *extent* of the documentation that can be attributed mainly to the growing cost of **data acquisition** and an upper limit for ways of analyzing the data.

As mentioned above, the extent of documentation essentially is determined by the number of data objects on the one hand, and the number of attributes recorded for each data object on the other hand. Documentation with many data objects and few attributes is called "broad" or **horizontal documentation** (examples: clinical **basic data set documentation**, and **cancer register**). Documentation with few data objects and many attributes is called "deep" or **vertical documentation** (examples: detailed findings of cardiac catheter examinations, and records of a **clinical study**).

Horizontal vs. vertical

Let us say that a data management system belongs to exactly one of the following classes:
Class D1:   Primarily vertical documentation
Class D2:   Primarily horizontal documentation
Class D3:   Mixture of vertical and horizontal documentation
Class D9:   Can't be assigned to one of the above

Classes

As you will have noticed, we have given no objective criteria for the assignment of the labels "horizontal" and "vertical." In borderline cases, different persons might make different assignments (as you will see later, this is a problem of **reliability**). What counts here is this: If you are planning a data management system, you have to limit its costs (in terms of time and money) to a degree that is justified by the results you get out of the system. In selecting one of the classes above, you will decide on whether you are saving with attributes or rather with data objects.

The data management system of PMC's neurological outpatient clinic contains very detailed information about the patients on the intensive care unit. For the other patients of the clinic, only general attributes like identifying data, diagnoses, and the length of stay are recorded. We therefore have vertical documentation for some object types (ICU patients), and horizontal documentation for others (normal patients): Again, a clear decision for the mixture class D3.

Example

Distinction by Directness

Data objects usually directly represent objects of the outer world, e.g., patients, diseases, **health care interventions**, etc. This is what we call direct documentation.

2.3.1.5

Direct documentation …

...vs. reference documentation

Sometimes, however, the objects represented are themselves data objects of another data management system, for example, journal articles and monographs in a library, or patient records in a record archive. In these cases, the focus of the data management system is on retrieving documents containing the desired information or medical knowledge. For this purpose, attributes describing documents and their location are recorded. In the case of journal articles, the attribute types could be the title of the paper, its authors and keywords, the journal's name and volume, and the library signature.

We then speak of **reference documentation**, or **indirect documentation**. Reference documentation can refer to documents being stored on different document carriers, which might themselves be located in different places.

Frequently mixed

Direct and reference documentation will often intersect. Take the basic data set documentation of a hospital as an example: Some questions (e.g., "Which patients, aged 80 years or above, died from leukemia?") can be answered directly; other questions (e.g., "How did the number of granulocytes develop during the last 2 weeks before the patient died?") can only be answered by following the documentation's link, or reference, to the laboratory **information system**.

Classes

Let us say that a data management system belongs to exactly one of the following classes:

Class R1: Primarily reference documentation
Class R2: Primarily direct documentation
Class R3: Mixture of direct and reference documentation
Class R9: Cannot be assigned to one of the above

Example

The information presented by the data management system of PMC's neurological outpatient clinic for the most part includes clinical facts about patients and elements of neurological knowledge. The system only gives some references to additional sources of medical knowledge. Thus, it can be classified as R2.

2.3.1.6 Distinction by Tools: Computer-Based or Conventional Systems

Features of computer-based tools

By using the computer as a tool, data management systems obtain a number of new qualities:

- Data can be retrieved and manipulated by different persons at the same time and from different places—given the necessary **communication links** and transaction control mechanisms.
- Data can be arranged (ordered, aggregated, transformed) for analysis in a way that is completely different from the way they have been recorded. Users are provided with different views on the data to meet their particular information requirements.
- **Computer systems** offer ample support for any data transformations (like aggregation, selection, reduction, combination, etc.) that might be needed for analysis.
- Data stored outside the data management system on another computer can be transferred into the data management system via a communication link. Establishing such a communication link between two systems may substantially reduce transmission errors and the time needed for data transfer.

There are many other features in which **computer-based data management systems** differ from not computer-based (or conventional) systems. One example is the different efforts connected with the activities of data acquisition, storage, retrieval, or output. Moreover, computer-based data management systems are usually standardized to a higher degree than conventional data management systems.

Let us say that a data management system belongs to exactly one of the following classes:

Classes

Class T1:   Computer-based
Class T2:   Conventional with computer support
Class T3:   Conventional (not computer-based)
Class T9:   Cannot be assigned to one of the above

The systems in class T2 are operated predominantly in a conventional manner. Only a few activities (e.g., the calculation of certain measures) are supported by a computer. In contrast, systems of class T1 rely fundamentally on the use of computers. As a matter of fact, almost all computer-based data management systems use conventional aids like, for example, **data entry** forms, printing of results, instruction leaflets, etc.

The data management system of PMC's neurological outpatient clinic is (almost) completely computer-based. It therefore falls under class T1.

Example

2.3.1.7   **Compositional Characterization of Clinical Data Management Systems**

In the last section, we introduced several criteria for the description of **medical data management systems**. Any system can be classified when using these criteria.

Example

In the data management system of Ploetzberg Medical Center the neurological outpatient clinic has been described as containing primarily clinical facts, aimed equally at patient-oriented as well as patient-group analyses, mainly standardized, mixture of vertical and horizontal documentation, primarily direct documentation, and computer-based. Using our formal **notation** this would be C1–U3–S3–D3–R2–T1.

Through the combination of the individual classes into an overall description of a data management system, you get a rather differentiated picture of its characteristics.

2.3.3   **Exercises**

Exercises 1–4

There are no exercises 1 to 4 in this chapter.

Exercise 5

Based on the attribute types and attribute values (referring to previous exercise 5), you have created documentation about hospitals including MHP. The aim was to give a brief description of each hospital and to indicate its diagnostic and therapeutic spectrum. Characterize (or design) the data management system for your hospital documentation on the basis of the criteria introduced in this chapter.

2.4   Medical Coding Systems

To find specific pieces of information within documentation, it is often necessary to use **documentary language**. To put it into simple terms, you need a set of keywords (or **authorized terms**) and rules for their application. If documentary languages are meant to cover a relevant part of medical reality, the authorized terms must be ordered systematically (i.e., the language must be based on a **concept system**); otherwise, it would be too unwieldy to work with. In that case, we call the documentary language a **coding system**. In the medical field, for instance, coding systems are common to document diagnoses and therapies.

What will you learn?

In this chapter you will learn
- what documentary languages or coding systems are good for in clinical data management systems, and when you shouldn't use them.
- the basic types of coding systems and the kinds of tasks they may support.

As you read through this chapter, refer to a copy (or have a look at the online version) of concrete coding systems and try to reflect on how the discussion pertains to a practical example.

Coding Systems: Why Do We Need Them?

2.4.1

Problems

Medical statements (e.g., about the diagnosis of a patient) can be made in various ways: a particular level of detail may be chosen; for every concept, one out of several synonymous labels may be selected; every term may have more than one possible spelling; and the whole statement may be structured according to the author's preferences. This freedom of expression can cause certain problems in subsequent **data analysis**:
- The retrieval of particular data objects is harder and less reliable if you don't know the terms and writing style used in their acquisition. The same diagnosis can be termed as, for example, a "liver rupture," a "hepatic laceration," or "hepatorrhexis."
- The usage of homonymous terms may lead to the selection of irrelevant data objects. For example, looking for "MI" in search of myocardial infarction may produce cases of mesenterial infection.
- It may be nearly impossible to count the frequency of certain similar objects (e.g., of certain diagnostic categories for administrative or for scientific purposes), because the terms used in the documentation do not indicate the degree of similarity between them. Two diagnoses, liver cirrhoses and subacute alcoholic hepatic dystrophy, may be regarded as similar in an administrative analysis, but as different in an epidemiological study.

Possible solutions

Documentary languages and coding systems restrict the variability of expression. To form statements, only authorized terms may be combined according to strict and simple rules. Usually, instead of an authorized term, a short and formal **code** is recorded, making statements shorter and easier to record. Following these restrictions, many of the difficulties mentioned above are avoided. To record the diagnosis of acute appendicitis, for example, you might have to use the code 540, which stands for the (preferred) authorized term "appendicitis, acute." The **preferred terms** will be used in analyses instead of the code to make them more readable.

On the other hand, one can think of many questions that cannot be answered precisely with such limited possibilities of expression. Especially decisions on the patient's care must include relevant detail, often recorded in free text form (e.g., whether the appendicitis was accompanied by a perforation or a peritonitis).

2.4.2   What Is a Coding System?

Orders the set of terms...

As we have said, a documentary language provides a set of authorized terms. This set is possibly very large and cannot be handled as a simple list, for example the set of all surgical procedures. Thus, an attempt is made to bring the authorized terms into a clear, often hierarchical, order.

...by ordering the concepts

Actually, the terms aren't ordered (except alphabetically), but the concepts they label are. In doing so, the documentary language is backed by a concept system. Surgical procedures, for example, can be divided into operations on the nervous system, on the abdomen, on the organs of the chest, on the blood vessels, etc. Operations on organs of the chest can be subdivided into operations on the heart, on the lung, etc., ending up with the distinction between a valvotomy of the left atrioventricular valve and a valvotomy of the aortic valve.

Coding system

A documentary language that is based on a concept system is called a coding system. With the help of an adequate coding system, the correct code for every medical fact (e.g., a surgical procedure) should quickly and reliably be accessible, if the necessary knowledge of the subject is at hand.

Thesaurus

In many cases it is helpful if the coding system also points out unauthorized terms, which are frequently used synonymously with an authorized term. The unauthorized term "Conn's syndrome," for example, might point you to the authorized term "primary hyperaldosteronism" and the corresponding code, 255.1. A coding system that is enhanced by terminological information like this is often called a thesaurus.

2.4.3   Classifications and Nomenclatures

Introduction

In planning a data management system, you must decide for every attribute if you should apply a coding system for the objectives of the system, and if it's better to choose a classification or a **nomenclature**.

To help you understand the advantages and disadvantages of both basic types of coding systems, we will introduce them in the following paragraphs and give some examples from the medical field.

Classifications

Classifications (also: classification systems) are coding systems founded on the principle of constructing classes. Classes form an aggregation of concepts that match in (at least) one **classifying attribute**. For example, all diseases with the classifying attributes of an inflammation of the myocardium as well as of an infectious etiology may be aggregated to the class "infectious myocarditis."

You can think of a class as a container for objects having this particular attribute. In the example above, this could be all discharge diagnoses of a health care institution involving infectious myocarditis.

The classes of a classification should cover the relevant domain completely and their contents should not overlap. Each object has to be assigned to exactly one class. When this is done the object is classified. The diagnosis of septic myocarditis, for example, might be assigned to the class "infectious myocarditis" mentioned above.

For the sake of brevity as well as of language independence (if you have editions of the classification in different languages), each class is provided with a code. This could be "357" for infectious myocarditis—"3.." denoting diseases of the cardiovascular system and "35.." an acute inflammation of the heart. The hierarchy expressed in this **coding** example is a typical construction principle of larger classifications.

Now, to document a medical fact, all you have to do is to find out the appropriate class (put it in the right "container") and record the class's code. This is what we call coding a medical fact.

Classifications are useful in those cases where documentation is used
- for patient-group analyses (e.g., to find out the frequency of cases of infectious myocarditis in the PMC during the last year);
- to find out all objects that are similar in a certain respect (for example, all patients of the PMC having had an extended hemicolectomy).

Classifying corresponds to the presentation of attribute values on a nominal scale (see level of measurement)—an important prerequisite for the use of statistical methods to analyze the class frequencies observed. The results of this analysis may be compared read-

2.4.3.1
Classes and classifying attributes

Complete and exhaustive

Coding

Application

Analysis of frequencies

Granularity

ily with the results of other institutions, as long as they are using the same classification system.

The usefulness of a classification essentially depends on the assumption that the objects aggregated in a class are equivalent with regard to the aspired analysis. If you want to distinguish, for example, hemicolectomies including a preternatural anus from those without, then the class "extended hemicolectomy" is too coarse for that purpose.

Forms

The structure of a classification can exhibit certain peculiarities (see also the examples in the next section):

Hierarchy

- The classes of a hierarchical classification are related exclusively either in a generic or in a **partitive** way, i.e., the subordinate concept, or class, in the hierarchy is either a specialization, or a part of the superordinate concept.

Monohierarchy vs. polyhierarchy

- In a monohierarchical classification, there is exactly one superordinate class to every class (except the topmost, or "root" of the hierarchy). In contrast, polyhierarchical classifications allow classes to be subordinated to more than one class, which results in several, overlying hierarchies.

Multiple axes or dimensions

- **Multiaxial classifications** (or **multidimensional classifications**) consist of two or more independent partial classifications. Here, a classifying attribute for each **axis** is needed, describing an object within different **semantic dimensions**. The object is classified in each axis separately.

Typical axes, or dimensions, you will find in multiaxial disease classifications are etiology, topography, and pathology. The partial classifications may themselves be structured hierarchically. In this case, you can think of an axis as a separate branch, or sub-tree, of the hierarchy.

Examples

A simple, monoaxial, and monohierarchical classification of diagnoses is as follows:

D1 Disorders of fat metabolism
    D11 Hyperlipidemia
    D12 Lipoproteinemia
        D121 Tangier Disease
        D122 A-Beta-lipoproteinemia
        D123 Other lipoproteinemia
    D13 Other disorders of fat metabolism

D2 Disorders of carbohydrate metabolism
    ...

An additional axis for etiology could contain the classes
A1 nutritional
A2 congenital
A3 mixed or other etiology

Together with the first axis (what would be its semantic dimension?), it forms a two-axial classification (see multiaxial classification). Hyperlipidemia caused by dietary habits would be coded as A1-D11.

If you find one class (e.g., viral menigitis) subordinate to two or more different superordinate classes (e.g., neurological diseases as well as viral diseases) you are dealing with a polyhierarchical classification.

Checklist: Classification

- Classifications consist of classes that should not overlap and that should completely cover the relevant domain completely. To achieve **completeness**, all hierarchical levels should include a class for "other"; however, this class will contain little information.
- Classifications of real-life complexity are usually structured hierarchically. You should distinguish between mono- and polyhierarchical classifications.
- A multiaxial classification originates by dividing a classification's concept system into several independent semantic dimensions.
- Assigning an object to exactly one class is called classifying, assigning the class's code to the object (which includes classifying) and recording it is called coding. Classification rules can help to find the right class.
- Classifying always leads to a loss of information (you focus on similarities to other objects in a class and neglect the differences); on the other hand, it enables patient-group analyses as well as the complete retrieval of similar objects.
- To answer the question whether a classification is good or bad, you have to know what kind of analysis you want to do. You need to determine whether it is appropriate or not.

Checklist

Nomenclatures

Basically, a nomenclature is no more than a systematic compilation of authorized terms for a certain documentation task. Due to their systematic structure and the provision of codes, nomenclatures usually take the form of coding systems. Additionally, the

2.4.3.2

Nomenclature, coding system, thesaurus

authorized terms may be complemented by definitions, synonymous terms, and other terminological notes; in that case, the nomenclature takes the form of a thesaurus.

Indexing with descriptors

A nomenclature is used to *mark* objects by assigning them all authorized terms (often called **descriptors**) that apply. We say that an object is **indexed**. In contrast to classifications, the concepts labeled by the descriptor may overlap. Moreover, an object is usually indexed with more than one descriptor.

If an object is not indexed completely, i.e., not all appropriate descriptors have been selected, there will be problems in retrieving the data object reliably. For example, if you have recorded the descriptor "localization: head" in documentation of pain symptoms, but have forgotten to record "characteristic: throbbing," you will miss the patient in a retrieval of all patients suffering a throbbing headache.

Coding

For the sake of brevity as well as for language independence, the authorized terms of a nomenclature are usually provided with a code. As for classifications, assigning a code is called coding.

Application

Nomenclatures are useful in those cases where documentation is used to retrieve the data on objects with a particular combination of attributes (e.g., all patients having had a meniscectomy under epidural anesthesia), and also to let computer programs process the information about objects (e.g., to translate it into another language, to warn of contraindications, or to suggest a treatment).

Retrieval quality

To measure the quality of the result of a specific retrieval, you have to check
- whether all relevant cases or patients have been retrieved, and
- whether the retrieved patients are all relevant.

Later we will introduce the measures of **precision** and **recall** for this purpose. These **quality indicators** are essential for the usefulness of a nomenclature; to a great degree, they are determined by how precisely relevant object features are expressed by the descriptors of the nomenclature. For example, if you only have the descriptors "operation on the knee" and "local anaesthesia" to index a meniscectomy under epidural, there might be too many irrelevant retrieval results for the question above.

Forms

Just like classifications, nomenclatures can have different constructions:

Hierarchy
- For easier orientation, extensive nomenclatures can exhibit hierarchical structures (i.e., can be based on a **hierarchical concept system**).

- Dividing the set of authorized terms into several semantic dimensions will lead to **multiaxial nomenclatures**. By checking the dimensions one after the other for applicable descriptors, the completeness of indexing is improved. Moreover, the reduced complexity serves the user with better orientation. In contrast to multiaxial classifications (where you have to choose exactly one class in every axis), you may well assign several descriptors per axis to one object. Multiple axes or dimensions
- In this context, a **list of descriptors** constitutes a simple, **monoaxial nomenclature**. List of descriptors

Imagine this list of descriptors for the localization of pain: **Examples**
L1 Head
L2 Back
L3 Extremities
L4 Joints

Assuming a hierarchical construction, this is a possible subdivision:
L1 Head
    L11 Face
    L12 Forehead
    L13 Temples
    L14 Skull

By adding another partial nomenclature for the quality of pain, a two-axial nomenclature emerges:
Q1 dull, pressing
Q2 burning, hot
Q3 stabbing, searing
Q4 tearing

A stabbing, hot pain at the wrist would be coded as (L3, L4, Q2, Q3). A dull pain at the forehead and a pressing pain at the temples would be two separate facts: (L12, Q1) and (L13, Q1).

Checklist: Nomenclature
Checklist

- Nomenclatures are systematically compiled sets of authorized terms or descriptors for a specific documentation task. As for classifications, rules can improve clarity.
- In contrast to classifications, the aim of a nomenclature is not to assign objects to categories but to describe them unambiguously and precisely in order to make them retrievable and processable.
- A nomenclature can be a simple alphabetical list of descriptors, or it can provide hierarchical structures to aid orientation.

- Dividing the set of authorized terms into different semantic dimensions creates a multiaxial nomenclature. Unlike with classifications, multiaxiality does not extend expressional power, but it facilitates handling.
- To mark an object with one or more descriptors is called indexing; to select the descriptors' codes and record them (which includes indexing) is called coding.
- To answer the question whether a nomenclature is good or bad, you have to know what kind of service it is meant to provide and whether it is appropriate or not.

2.4.3.3 Hybrid Forms of Classifications and Nomenclatures

One tool for all tasks

Every coding system must be understood and mastered by its users. Typical coding systems for diseases or therapies fill several volumes. Once people are used to a particular coding system, they want to use it for purposes it was not designed for originally. In this situation, you should keep two points in mind:

A nomenclature to classify

- To be able to use a nomenclature to classify objects "on the side," there are two prerequisites: First, you need a classification that covers the field completely and whose classes do not overlap. Second, a mapping function must be developed that maps every sensible combination of descriptors to exactly one class of the classification. This is not easy since there might be huge number of possible combinations that must be rechecked with every modification of the nomenclature. Moreover, the complete indexing of every object is difficult to ensure, so that the accuracy of class assignment might substantially depend on the care of the indexing person.

A classification to index

- To be able to use a classification to index objects, a way must be found to assign more than one class name as descriptors to one object. For example, the diagnosis of mumps with hepatitis could be classified as "mumps with complications-†" and additionally assigned the descriptor "hepatitis in viral diseases-*." The † symbol denotes a descriptor that is also the name of the assigned class; the * symbol denotes a supplementary descriptor without class quality. Clear rules as to which descriptor is to be marked with the † or the * symbol are necessary.

Even if this procedure seems to be quite popular—e.g., with editorial boards of international coding systems—it is only a makeshift, since there is limited usefulness of coding systems for tasks requiring a different structure.

A Simple Example

The Coding Systems

To record discharge diagnoses, the neurological department of the Ploetzberg Medical Center and Medical School (PMC) has two coding systems: a classification and a nomenclature.

This is an excerpt from the classification

A classification

K433.- Occlusion or stenosis of precerebral arteries
    K433.0 A. basilaris
    K433.1 A. carotis
    K433.8 Occlusion or stenosis of other precerebral arteries
...

This is an excerpt of the two-axial nomenclature:

A nomenclature

Axis 1: Morphology	Axis 2: Topography
...	...
M341- Stenosis	T45- Precerebral arteries
M3411 Stenosis due to calci-	T4511 A. carotis comm. dex.
fication	T4512 A. carotis comm. sin.
...	...
M351- Thrombosis	
M3511 Obturating thrombus	
...	

At the neurological department, the classification is used to tabulate the frequency of the diseases that were diagnosed over time. The nomenclature is intended to facilitate the retrieval of cases with certain attributes.

A Diagnosis

A diagnosis

The disease of a patient is diagnosed as "stenosis of the left arteria carotis communis with obstructive thrombosis."

Using the coding system above, the diagnosis can be indexed and classified as follows:

Classification: K433.1 (Occlusion or stenosis of the A. carotis)

Indexing: M3511 (Obturating thrombus)
                M3411 (Stenosis due to calcification)
                T4512 (A. carotis comm. sin.)

Coding the diagnoses of all patients of a health care institution in this way will enable the data management system to answer various questions. In the next paragraphs, we will give two typical examples.

Typical use of a classification

Typical Use of a Classification

Classifications are intended to describe the set of all objects aggregated in one class, e.g., as an answer to the question

Question 1: How many patients with the diagnoses falling into the class "occlusion or stenosis of the precerebral arteries" (K433.-) have been treated in our institution in the previous year?

Using a nomenclature?

This information could also be obtained using the indexed diagnoses. You would have to look for the simultaneous appearance of the code T45- (precerebral arteries) and the codes M351- (thrombus) or M341- (stenosis). The problem is, however, to guarantee that
- topography and morphology are indexed completely for all patients;
- all relevant indices are taken into account in the query;
- a patient is not counted more than once (this would particularly bias the comparison of class frequencies).

Typical use of a nomenclature

Typical Use of a Nomenclature

Nomenclatures are designed for the retrieval of data objects using differentiated, flexibly formulated criteria, e.g., as an answer to the following question:

Question 2: Who are the patients that suffered from a thrombosis of the arteria carotis communis without having a stenosis?

To answer this question, you would look for the simultaneous appearance of the codes M351- (thrombus) and T451- (A. carotis comm.), but without the code M341- (stenosis).

Using a classification?

This analysis is hardly possible when using the classified diagnoses because patients with and without stenosis belong to the same class, and the parts of the a. carotis are not differentiated. Using a classification for retrieval, the search criteria are limited to the classifying attributes. In our case, you could search, for example, for all cases with an occlusion or with a stenosis of the arteria carotis (K433.1) and subsequently browse the patient records to determine whether the patient had a thrombosis without stenosis at the a. carotis comm.

A Few Additional Remarks

- We previously introduced the multiaxial classification. Reconsider the characteristics of medical data management systems in section 2.3.1 against this background.
- We have already mentioned it but we want to say it again: No documentary language, or coding system, can be designed so concisely that it provides exactly one possible representation for any given medical fact. Classifications must be augmented and supported by additional rules, regulating, for example, that the disease class "inflammation of the lacrimal canal" does not apply to neonatal dacryosystitis, as there is a dedicated class "Dacryocystitis neonatorum" for that diagnosis.
- We have said that documentary languages can take on the form of a thesaurus by specifying additional terminological information. Therefore, you should be quite familiar with the Thesaurus of Medical Documentation (Chapter 11).

Exercises

What is the use of medical coding systems?

Exercise 1

Classifications and nomenclatures: Define these concepts. What are they used for? What are the differences?

Exercise 2

State the general advantages and disadvantages of multiaxial classifications as compared to **monoaxial classifications**.

Exercise 3

Data management system, coding system, concept system and thesaurus: Define these concepts. Describe the relationships between them. Give examples.

Exercise 4

To characterize the size and the range of services of the hospitals in your documentation referring to previous exercises 5, you probably used one or two, perhaps even more, classifications. If you haven't, you should do it now.

Exercise 5

In a discharge letter of the surgical department of the PMC, the following diagnosis is stated for patient Adams: "Carcinoma of the rectum, height 15 cm; chronic bronchitis."

Exercise 6

There is a nomenclature of diseases:

Topography		Morphology		
T260	Bronchus	M001	Acute progression	
T270	Bronchiolus	...		
...		M400	Inflammation	
T680	(Intestinum) rectum	...		
T681	Tunica mucosa recti	M800	Tumor	
...			M801	Benign tumor
T690	Anus		M802	Tumor with unknown malignity
...			M803	Malignant tumor
		...		

Index the diagnoses of Mr. Adams. Is it necessary to regard the two diagnoses in isolation?

Exercise 7

Additionally, there is a classification of diseases at your disposal. Here is an excerpt:

...

K154.- Malignant neoplasm of the rectum and the anus
    K154.1 Malignant neoplasm of the rectum
    K154.2 Malignant neoplasm of the anal canal
    K154.3 Malignant neoplasm of the anus
        exclusive: perianal skin → K172.5

...

    K172.5 Malignant melanoma of the skin of the trunk

...

K491.- Chronic bronchitis
    K491.1 Simple chronic bronchitis
    K491.2 Obstructive chronic bronchitis
    K491.3 Other forms of chronic bronchitis
    K491.9 Chronic bronchitis, not otherwise specified (n.o.s.)

...

Classify the diagnoses of Mr. Adams ("carcinoma of the rectum, height 15 cm; chronic bronchitis").

Important Medical Coding Systems   3

In this chapter we introduce important medical **coding systems**. There are many other systems, some of which are very common in their specialized fields. For specific research projects, dedicated coding systems must be developed. As even the most specialized systems usually serve multiple purposes, some of them externally motivated, they should be designed as an extension to a more general, standard coding system.

While you read this chapter, refer to a coding system, available on the Internet or at libraries.

Introduction

In this chapter you will learn about some important medical **concept systems**. You can familiarize yourself with
- the essential points of their origin;
- their basic structure;
- their application principles.

What will you learn?

International Classification of Diseases (ICD)   3.1

The **International Classification of Diseases** (ICD) is the most important diagnostic **classification** system. It is globally accepted and has been published by the World Health Organization (WHO) since its 6th revision in 1946.

Introduction

The ICD is used for WHO's global statistics of mortality and morbidity (go to http://www.who.int/whosis) and for a multitude of national, regional, and organizational purposes. These include health reporting, reimbursement for medical services, and health **care quality** control. Because of the ICD's comparatively coarse granularity, it has few applications in clinical research.

The foundations of the ICD were laid by William Farr in 1855 and extended by Jacques Bertillon, who presented his "International List of Causes of Death" in 1893. The list was adopted by the International Statistical Institute (ISI) and recommended for international use in 1899. There was a decision to revise it every 10 years. When the WHO took on the publication responsibility of the 6th revision conference in 1946, functionality was extended from reporting only on mortality to reporting on morbidity as well. The list was then renamed "International Classification of Diseases and Causes of Death." In 1989, the 10th revision of the ICD (ICD-10) was approved.

Origin

Most countries in the world have adopted the 10th revision of the ICD for their official reporting procedures or have started the transition process from the 9th revision.

3.1.1   The 10th Revision (ICD-10)

Structure and code

The "International Statistical Classification of Diseases and Related Health Problems," tenth revision (ICD-10), is a monoaxial and monohierarchical classification with a four- to five-digit **code**.

In certain application areas, only the first three digits of the code are used, but for most purposes the finer granularity of the fourth digit is needed. There are a number of subclasses or specializations labeled by a fifth digit.

The code is alphanumeric: the first character is a letter, followed by two to four figures; the fourth digit is separated by a decimal point.

The hierarchy of the ICD-10 is represented in
- 21 disease chapters (e.g., Chapter IV: Endocrine, Nutritional, and Metabolic Diseases; see Table 3.1),
- 261 disease groups (e.g., group E10-E14: diabetes mellitus),
- about 2000 three-digit disease **classes** (e.g., class E10: insulin-dependent diabetes mellitus),
- more than 12,000 four-digit disease classes (e.g., class E10.1: insulin-dependent diabetes mellitus with ketoacidosis).

Special characteristics

By introducing an alphanumerical code, the number of possible classes has been expanded considerably compared with the ICD-9, which had a strictly numerical **notation**. The codes U50 to U99 have been reserved for research purposes.

Classes have been constructed mainly on the basis of statistical criteria, like the **prevalence** of a disease.

There is no common **semantic dimension** underlying the classification's hierarchy: Most chapters are **defined** according to the body systems (or topography), some according to etiology, and some according to pathology (see Table 3.1).

There are descriptions of a disease that might be related to more than one class of the classification. To assign them reproducibly to exactly one class, the ICD gives classification rules with extensive inclusion and exclusion criteria. For example, acute bronchitis usually is coded as a four-digit specialization of J20 (acute bronchitis), except when it is an allergic reaction, which has to be coded under J45 (asthma).

Table 3.1 Disease chapters of the ICD-10.

Chapter	Title	Code (3-dig.)
I	Certain infectious and parasitic diseases	A00-B99
II	Neoplasms	C00-D48
III	Diseases of the blood and blood-forming organs and certain disorders involving the immune mechanism	D50-D89
IV	Endocrine, nutritional and metabolic diseases	E00-E90
V	Mental and behavioral disorders	F00-F99
VI	Diseases of the nervous system	G00-G99
VII	Diseases of the eye and adnexa	H00-H59
VIII	Diseases of the ear and mastoid process	H60-H95
IX	Diseases of the circulatory system	I00-I99
X	Diseases of the respiratory system	J00-J99
XI	Diseases of the digestive system	K00-K93
XII	Diseases of the skin and subcutaneous tissue	L00-L99
XIII	Diseases of the musculoskeletal system and connective tissue	M00-M99
XIV	Diseases of the genitourinary system	N00-N99
XV	Pregnancy, childbirth, and the puerperium	O00-O99
XVI	Certain conditions originating in the perinatal period	P00-P96
XVII	Congenital malformations, deformations, and chromosomal abnormalities	Q00-Q99
XVIII	Symptoms, signs, and abnormal clinical and laboratory findings, not elsewhere classified	R00-R99
XIX	Injury, poisoning, and certain other consequences of external causes	S00-T98
XX	External causes of morbidity and mortality	V01-Y98
XXI	Factors influencing health status and contact with health services	Z00-Z99

The ICD usually requires the basic disease process to be **classified**. In some cases, localized manifestations of that process may be coded additionally. The basic disease code then is marked with a dagger (†), and the localized manifestation with an asterisk (*). For example, meningitis as a complication of rubella is coded as B06.0† (rubella with neurological complications) and G02.0* (meningitis due to viral infections).

Here, the * code can be used to retrieve cases of meningitis, but will be ignored in analyses that require each case to be counted only once.

Example

Extract from the tabular section of the ICD-10:

Chapter XI: Diseases of the digestive system (K00–K93)
Excl.   Congenital malformations, deformations, and chromosomal ab-
        normalities (Q00–Q99)
        Certain infectious and parasitic diseases (A00–B99)
        Certain conditions originating in the perinatal period (P00–P96)
[...]
**Diseases of esophagus, stomach, and duodenum
(K20-K31)**
Excl.   Diaphragmatic hernia (K44.-)
[...]
K22   **Other diseases of esophagus**
           Excl. Esophageal varices (I85.-)

K22.0   **Achalasia of cardia**
        Incl. Achalasia n.o.s.
               dilatation of esophagus
        Exkl. Congenital dilatation of esophagus (Q39.5)
K22.1   **Ulcer of esophagus**
[...]

3.1.2   Extensions to the ICD

**Why
extensions?**

The ICD is a very general classification of diseases, created from
the global, mortality-oriented perspective of the WHO. Many
medical specialties found it to be insufficient for their scientific or
reporting purposes. Consequently, they made extensions to the
ICD in **terms** of subclasses, covering their area of interest in finer
granularity. Among others, there are ICD extensions in the fields
of ophthalmology, dermatology, pediatrics, neurology, oncology,
orthopedics, and rheumatology. Ideally, the extensions are designed in a way that allows every specialized class to be reduced
unambiguously and automatically to its basic ICD class.

ICD-CM

While the United States applies the ICD for its mortality statistics,
a clinical modification (ICD-CM) has been developed that extends,
modifies, and clarifies the ICD **concepts** to meet the terminological and organizational requirements of the health care setting. In
the U.S., the ICD-CM is used for morbidity statistics, health sur-
veys, and hospital utilization reviews. It has been translated into
French, Dutch, Spanish, and Portuguese.
The transition from revision 9 (ICD-9-CM) to revision 10 (ICD-
10-CM) is planned for the end of 2001.

ICD-O

In 1976, the WHO first published the International Classification
of Diseases for Oncology, ICD-O. ICD-O's topography code ex-

tends the neoplasms section of ICD's Chapter II to describe the site of a tumor's origin. The morphology code describes the characteristics of the tumor itself, including its cell type and biological activity.

Procedure Classifications

The goal of investigating costs and performance guides the efforts to classify **health care interventions**, or procedures. This is why the first approaches to procedure classifications concentrated on costly interventions like operations and machine-aided diagnosis.

International Classification of Procedures in Medicine (ICPM)

The WHO's **International Classification of Procedures in Medicine** (ICPM) has been the basis for a number of medical procedure classification systems. In extended and modified forms, it constitutes a regular part of the health reporting and financing procedures in many countries of the world.

In 1978, WHO published the ICPM for research purposes. The classification has fairly coarse granularity. No revision has been offered by the WHO despite the continuously evolving spectrum of medical procedures. So the WHO's ICPM provided only a framework for national extensions and updates.

In the Netherlands and in Germany, extended versions of the ICPM have been developed (ICPM-DE, the Dutch Extension, and OPS301, the German Surgical Procedure Codes). Both classifications are mandatory in the respective countries for reimbursement and administration procedures in the inpatient sector.
The U.S. ICD-9-CM volume 3 procedure classification is based on the surgical procedures chapter of the ICPM. Note that volume 3 of the ICD-9-CM, classifying procedures rather than diseases, has nothing to do with the WHO's ICD-9.
In the ICD-10-CM, however, the procedural part will be replaced by a completely new coding system, the ICD-10-PCS, or Procedure Coding System (see next section).

Example: ICD-9-CM Procedure Classification

ICD-9-CM, together with its procedure classification in volume 3, is published and annually revised by the U.S. National Center for Health Statistics (NCHS) and the Health care Financing Administration (HCFA). It is originally based on the surgical procedures chapter of the ICPM but has been adopted since to reflect clinical practice in the U.S. hospital sector.

ICD-9-CM, volume 3, forms a **monoaxial classification**.

- It is divided into 16 chapters (e.g., 4: Operations on the Ear; see Table 3.2). Most of the procedures are surgical operations, but there is one chapter on miscellaneous diagnostic and therapeutic procedures, containing, for example, radiological diagnostics and physiotherapeutic procedures.
- Each chapter contains up to 13 two-digit procedure groups (e.g., 19: reconstructive operations on middle ear).
- Each procedure group contains up to 9 three-digit procedures (e.g., 19.1: Stapedectomy), possibly further specified by a fourth digit (e.g., 19.11: Stapedectomy with incus replacement).

Code

The code is numeric, with the first two digits representing the procedure group and the third and possibly fourth digit, separated by a decimal point, representing the procedure and its specification. "9" as the third or the fourth digit indicates "not otherwise specified (n.o.s.) procedures" in the given superclass.

Further characteristics

The structure of the classification is topographically oriented; there is no division by medical specialties.

To support the accurate use of the classification, inclusion and exclusion criteria have been formulated as well as further usage notes (see the following example).

Table 3.2 Chapters of ICD-9-CM, volume 3 (NCHS, Financial Year 1999).

Chapter	Title	Procedure Groups
1	Operations on the Nervous System	01-05
2	Operations on the Endocrine System	06-07
3	Operations on the Eye	08-16
4	Operations on the Ear	18-20
5	Operations on the Nose, Mouth, and Pharynx	21-29
6	Operations on the Respiratory System	30-34
7	Operations on the Cardiovascular System	35-39
8	Operations on the Hemic and Lymphatic System	40-41
9	Operations on the Digestive System	42-54
10	Operations on the Urinary System	55-59
11	Operations on the Male Genital Organs	60-64
12	Operations on the Female Genital Organs	65-71
13	Obstetrical Procedures	72-75
14	Operations on the Musculoskeletal System	76-84
15	Operations on the Integumentary System	85-86
16	Miscellaneous Diagnostic and Therapeutic Procedures	87-99

Extract from the tabular section of the ICD-9-CM, vol. 3
(NCHS, Financial Year 1999):

7. Operations on the Cardiovascular System (35-39)

35	Operations on valves and septa of heart

Includes: sternotomy (median) (transverse) as operative approach
         thoracotomy as operative approach
Code also cardiopulmonary bypass [extracorporeal circulation]
         [heart-lung machine] (39.61)

35.0   Closed heart valvotomy
Excludes: percutaneous (balloon) valvuloplasty (35.96)

   35.00   Closed heart valvotomy, unspecified valve
   35.01   Closed heart valvotomy, aortic valve
   35.02   Closed heart valvotomy, mitral valve
   35.03   Closed heart valvotomy, pulmonary valve
   35.04   Closed heart valvotomy, tricuspid valve

[…]

35.9   Other operations on valves and septa of heart
[…]

ICD-10-Procedure Coding System (ICD-10-PCS)

The ICD-10-Procedure Coding System (ICD-10-PCS) was devel-oped by 3M Health Information Systems starting in 1995 on behalf of the HCFA and will be introduced as volume 3 of the ICD-10-CM, together with the ICD-10 diagnosis classification (hence the acronym). Its development was initiated for the purpose of creating an accurate, unambiguous, expandable, and efficient coding sys-tem for all medical procedures. The development phase has been followed by an extensive testing and improvement process con-cluded in 2000.
Other countries are considering the introduction of ICD-10-PCS in their own health care systems.

ICD-10-PCS forms a **multiaxial classification**. The notation is alphanumeric (the letters I and O have been excluded to avoid confusion with the digits 1 and 0). There are seven characters per procedure code. The letter Z is used to indicate that a character is not applicable for a specific procedure.

Sections   - The coding system is divided into 16 sections, represented by the first character of the code (Table 3.3).

Table 3.3   Sections of the ICD-10-PCS (HCFA, Final Draft 1998, last updated 11/2000). The section's identifier provides the first digit of a procedure's seven-character code.

Identifier	Section
0	Medical and Surgical
1	Obstetrics
2	Placement
3	Administration
4	Measurement and Monitoring
5	Imaging
6	Nuclear Medicine
7	Radiation Oncology
8	Osteopathic
9	Rehabilitation and Diagnostic Audiology
B	Extracorporeal Assistance and Performance
C	Extracorporeal Therapies
D	Laboratory
F	Mental Health
G	Chiropractic
H	Miscellaneous

- The meaning of the other characters varies between sections. For the first two sections, 0 and 1, the character assignments are shown in Fig. 3.1.

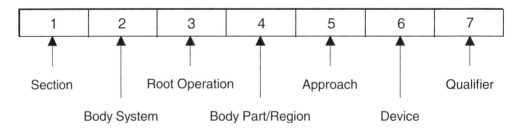

Fig. 3.1   PCS Character Assignment for the sections Medical and Surgical, and Obstetrics (HCFA, Final Draft 1998, last updated 11/2000).

Body system   - The body system, second character in 14 of the 16 sections, uses 31 generally accepted anatomical categories like central nervous system (0), upper arteries (3), eye (8), respiratory system (B), lower extremities (Z), etc.

Root operation   - The root operation, third character in 13 of the 16 sections, denotes the underlying objective of a procedure. All possible medical and surgical procedure can be reduced to only 30 root operations like bypass (1), dilation (7), excision (B), occlusion

(L), resection (T), or transplantation (Y). An explicit definition is provided with each root operation term.

- The body part/region specifies the anatomical part or region upon which the procedure is performed; the choice depends on the body system as well as the root operation indicated in the second and third characters. For example, in the heart and great vessels (2) body system, a drainage (9) root operation can be performed only on the body part pericardium (P), whereas a dilation (7) root operation can be performed on coronary arteries, pulmonary arteries and veins, heart valves, etc.

Body part / region

- The approach specifies the method by which the body part is reached or exposed in the procedure. There are approaches through the skin (open, percutaneous, percutaneous endoscopic, etc.), approaches through an orifice, or operations without an approach (e.g., skin excision or closed fracture reduction).

Approach

- Only those devices are stated that remain after completion of the procedure. Examples are drainage device, autograft, synthetic substitute.

Devices

- Qualifiers provide additional **information** on a procedure; they have a unique meaning for individual procedures.

Qualifier

Example procedure codes of the Medical and Surgical Procedures section (0):

Examples

097H1DZ   Ear, Nose, Sinus (9): Dilation (7): Eustachian Tube, right (H): Open Intraluminal (1): with Intraluminal Device (D): no qualifier (Z)

04100ZH   Lower Arteries (4): Bypass (1), Abdominal Aorta (0), Open (0): no device (Z): to Femoral Artery, right (H)

0KQ007Z   Muscles (K): Repair (Q): Head Muscles (0): Open (0) with Autograft (7): no qualifier (Z)

In other sections, some of the code's characters describe features relevant only to procedures in this section. Some examples:

Other characteristics

- In the administration Section (3), the sixth character denotes the substance administered, e.g., whole blood, anti-inflammatory, contrast agent, etc.

Substance

- In the measurement and monitoring section (4), the same character denotes the function that is measured or monitored, e.g., urinary flow, body temperature.

Function

- In the imaging section (5), the third character indicates the type of imaging, i.e., plain radiography, fluoroscopy, CT scan, MRI, and ultrasound.

Imaging type

Due to the multiaxial structure of the classification, **coding** must be a sequential process. Seven decisions have to be made, starting

Coding process

with the choice of the section, the body system, the root operation, and so on.

Index

To support the first three to four choices, an alphabetical **index** is provided for coders who have not yet "internalized" the systems structure and definitions. The index does not include eponyms.

Tabular listing

Once the first three characters are selected, the coder ends up in a tabular listing that provides all possible further choices on a single page (in most cases).

Further remarks

- In contrast to conventional classifications, like the ICD, the PCS system tries to avoid "not-elsewhere-classified (n.e.c.)" and "not-otherwise-specified (n.o.s.)" classes as much as possible to increase the specificity of coding.
- The multiaxial design enables high coding specificity at a moderate size of the classification system. The concise, even though sometimes unfamiliar, term definitions increase the accuracy of the results. On the one hand, these features greatly improve the results in finding cases where specific procedures have been performed. On the other hand, both features require a substantial training effort for those who code procedures.
- **Computer** support can significantly speed up the coding process, but it cannot eliminate the need for conscious choices made by the coder.
- Certain objectives of **data analysis**, like the comparison of institutions or the determination of case groups, require the **data** to be assigned to a reasonably small number of groups. Because of the high specificity of the PCS system, these groups have to be defined by a mapping procedure starting from all possible PCS codes. Once this procedure is defined, the grouping can be done automatically, as it is done in the Diagnosis-Related Groups (DRG) system. Every extension and modification to the PCS system, however, requires a modification of the mapping, and it indirectly changes the definition of the groups.

3.3 Systematized Nomenclature of Medicine (SNOMED)

Significance and purpose

The Systematized **Nomenclature** of Human and Veterinary Medicine (**SNOMED**) is the most important of general medical nomenclatures. SNOMED's purpose is to **label**, or index, medical statements in a way that covers their content as completely as possible. Thus, a **data management system** can produce retrieval results with high **recall** and **precision**. Very specific links to other collections of information or knowledge (e.g., case collections or literature databases) can be established. By using SNOMED's formal labels, specialized programs can support subsequent decisions in the process of clinical care.

Indexing with SNOMED produces a language-independent representation of a medical statement. Using translations of the same SNOMED version, a statement can be automatically translated into another language.

SNOMED developed from the Systematized Nomenclature of Pathology (SNOP) which was first published in 1965. Both nomenclatures are published by the College of American Pathologists (CAP).

Origin

The first version of SNOMED appeared in the U.S. in 1975 and was followed by a first revision in 1979 (SNOMED 2nd edition). Friedrich Wingert used this revision as a basis for his extended German version, which in turn influenced SNOMED International, or SNOMED III, published by CAP in 1993.

SNOMED International was translated into several languages and is being used in more than 30 countries worldwide.

In May 2000, CAP presented SNOMED Reference **Terminology** (SNOMED RT) as its most recent development. Moreover, CAP entered into an agreement with the U.K. National Health Service (NHS) to combine SNOMED RT with NHS's Clinical Terms, Version 3 (CTV3, or Read Codes) to form a comprehensive medical terminology, called SNOMED Clinical Terms (SNOMED CT).

SNOMED Reference Terminology (SNOMED RT)

3.3.1

SNOMED RT establishes a hierarchical system of clinical concepts that is divided into 12 root hierarchies or subhierarchies, describing different semantic dimensions (Table 3.4). As any medical statement may be labeled with concepts from several semantic dimensions, SNOMED RT can be said to be a **multiaxial nomenclature**. Additionally, a concept may have more than one predecessor in its root hierarchy (e.g., pneumococcal pneumonia is an infectious disease as well as a bacterial disease), which makes SNOMED RT a polyhierarchical nomenclature.

Structure

In SNOMED RT, every concept is identified by a strictly non-semantic numerical identifier. It contains no intrinsic information about a concept's position inside the overall system. Thus, problems with concepts that reside in multiple hierarchies are avoided. For external representation, an additional SNOMED identifier is stored with every concept. It has a two-part alphanumerical nota-

Code

tion: the first one or two characters identify the root hierarchy (e.g., T for topography or P for procedures). The second part of the notation consists of four to five characters identifying the concept itself (e.g., DA-00015—disorder: brain damage; F-D0922—biological function: neutrophil chemotaxis).

Hierarchies and relations

All hierarchies are based on typed relations between the concepts. Typically, these are generic ("is a") and **partitive** ("part-whole") relations. So, for example, in the topography hierarchy, the duodenum is part of the small intestine, which in turn is part of the digestive tract. In the disease hierarchy, arteritis is a vasculitis and is a disease of artery.

Concept explication

Relations can be used not only to build up hierarchies but also to explicate the meaning of higher level concepts. Concepts from the modifier/linkage hierarchy are used to "type" the relation.

Table 3.4 Root Hierarchies of SNOMED RT.
SOAP is an acronym for the structure of clinical progress notes suggested by Larry Weed: subjective, objective, assessment, plan.

Root hierarchy	Description
Diseases	
Findings, conclusions, and/or assessments	Disorders, clinical findings (by site, method, function); the S, O, and A of a SOAP note
Procedures	Plans, interventions, therapies, prescriptions, operations; the P of a SOAP note
Body structures - topography	Normal anatomical and topographical structures
Body structures - morphology	Abnormal structures (pathology and morphology)
Physical agents, activities, and/or forces	Causes of injury, devices, prostheses
Living organisms	Living organisms of etiological significance (bacteria, viruses, fungi, plants, animals)
Biological functions	Physiology and pathophysiology of disease processes, including abilities and properties
Occupations	An international occupational classification
Substances	Drugs, chemicals, and biological products of etiologic or therapeutic relevance
Modifiers/linkage terms and/or qualifiers	Context, modifiers, location, certainty, severity, course, time frames, staging, status, properties; linkage of concepts
Specimen	
Social context/demographics	

The disease concept of a ruptured ovarian cyst (D7-75111) can be defined as a disease (DF-00000) which **Example**
– has morphology (G-C480) rupture (M-14400) and
– has morphology (G-C480) cyst (M-33400) and
– has topography (G-C006) ovary (T-87000).

This mechanism (or grammar) is also used to represent clinical statements made in the course of a patient's care. **Clinical statements**

The clinical statement "Malignant carcinoid tumor of rectum with carcinoid syndrome" may be represented as: **Examples**
  (DF-000000) disease
  and (G-C006 T-59600) has topography rectum
  and (G-C480 M-82413) has morphology carcinoid tumor, malignant
  and (G-C016 DB-00050) associated with carcinoid syndrome

The statement "Crushing substernal chest pain radiating to the left arm" would be expressed as:
  (F-37070) crushing chest pain
  and (F-37022) substernal chest pain
  and (G-C040 T-D8220) radiating to left arm.

Using other "Linkage" concepts, SNOMED expressions may represent complex clinical statements combining, for example, a disease with its etiology, the diagnostic and therapeutic procedures, and complications of these procedures.

Excerpt from the *Findings* dimension of SNOMED RT: **Examples**

F-18001 Normal gait
F-18002 Gait abnormality
F-18003 Difficulty walking
F-18070 Shuffling gait
F-18080 Athetotic gait
F-180A0 Staggering gait
F-180B0 Cerebellar gait
F-180C0 Ataxic gait

Excerpt from the *Procedures* dimension of SNOMED RT:

P1-5B800 Repair of liver
P1-5B806 Marsupialization of cyst or abscess of liver
P1-5B810 Suture of liver
P1-5B812 Complex hepatorrhaphy
P1-5B814 Complex hepatorrhaphy with hepatic artery ligation
P1-5B816 Hepatorrhaphy with common duct or gallbladder drainage
P1-5B830 Hepatopexy

Concepts vs. terms

Every concept in SNOMED is associated with one **preferred term** and possibly with one or more **synonymous terms**, facilitating usage variations and language translation.

Scope

SNOMED RT contains more than 120,000 concepts and 190,000 terms. More than 340,000 relationships between concepts have been explicitly defined. Concepts, descriptions (or terms), and relationships are the three core relational tables in which SNOMED RT is delivered.

Mappings to ICD-9-CM and ICD-O

Some 24,000 SNOMED concepts (from the disease and findings hierarchies) have been mapped to ICD-9-CM classes. Roughly a third of these mappings are one-to-one matches; most of the others map a narrower SNOMED concept to a broader ICD-9-CM class. Topographical and morphological concepts have been mapped to the ICD-O. With these mappings, a carefully derived SNOMED representation of a clinical statement may automatically produce valid ICD codes for statistical or billing purposes.

3.3.2   SNOMED Clinical Terminology (SNOMED CT)

SNOMED RT + Read Codes

SNOMED Clinical Terms (SNOMED CT) is a joint effort of the CAP and the U.K.'s NHS. Announced in April 1999, SNOMED CT combines SNOMED RT and NHS's Clinical Terms version 3 (CTV3, the Read Codes), an extensive and successful terminology in the U.K. The goals of the cooperation are to share expertise and development costs, to cross-evaluate the systems, to draw on economies of scale, and to introduce an international perspective.

Unified terminology

The originators see SNOMED CT as a single unified terminology, building the foundation of the electronic medical record and supporting all health care professions in providing good clinical care. Additionally, the system is expected to support a number of secondary purposes (e.g., statistical and billing) and provide a basic building block for worldwide clinical **communication**.

Scope

With the integration of CTV3, SNOMED CT has grown to more than 320,000 concepts, 800,000 descriptions, or terms, and about 1 million explicit relationships. Like SNOMED RT, there are three core relational tables: concepts, descriptions (or terms), and relationships. They are related to each other as shown in Fig. 3.2, and supplemented by tables for subset definitions, for change management, and for mappings to other terminologies (e.g., ICD-10).

SNOMED CT has been released in February 2002. In the U.K., every computerized clinical **information system** is expected to implement SNOMED CT by April 2003.

Version 1 released

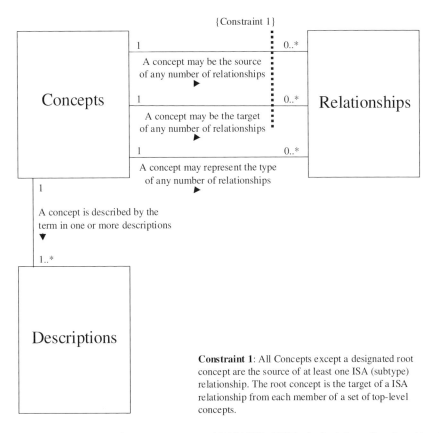

Fig. 3.2   The SNOMED CT core structure (SNOMED CT Technical Specification, Version 19, October 2000). Note that
      – the type of a relationship is itself a concept;
      – every concept is part of a generic ("is a") hierarchy.

The TNM Classification of Malignant Tumors   3.4

The **TNM system** provides a standardized classification of the anatomical extension of malignant tumor diseases, or of their staging, as it is commonly called. TNM serves as an extension of the topographical and histological description of tumors on the basis of the ICD-O, the oncological add-on classification to the ICD.

Purpose

In 1953, the International Union against Cancer (UICC) and the International Commission on Stage-Grouping in Cancer and Presentation of the Results of Treatment of Cancer agreed on a general

Origin

method to classify the extent of malignant tumors. This method, the TNM system, was developed by Pierre Denoix, starting in 1943.

In the course of the following years, the UICC Committee on Clinical Stage Classification and Applied Statistics worked out a number of suggestions for the classification of tumor locations and gathered them in a manual that was published in 1968. The manual has been translated into 11 languages.

The fifth and most recent English edition was published in 1997.

3.4.1   Structure

Basic classification

The extent of a (previously specified) tumor disease is indicated by numbers assigned to each of three components:

T (tumor)	–	Extension of the primary tumor: T0 to T4;
N (nodule)	–	Existence and spread of lymph node metastases: N0 to N3;
M (metastasis)	–	Existence of distant metastases: M0 or M1.

Coding examples: T2N1M0, T3N1MX (X for 'not assessable').

With this, the TNM system basically forms a three-axial classification.

Classification rules

Detailed rules of classification specify which number, or class, has to be assigned in each of the three **axes**, or dimensions. The purpose is to ensure **reliability** of coding. The rules do not apply generally, but only in relation to a particular *anatomical region*, indicated by a topographical code of the ICD-O. The ICD-O's topographical section extends the neoplasms chapter of the ICD-10. An example:

Example

Definition of stage T2 of a larynx tumor:
Supraglottis (ICD-O topography C32.1):
  T2: Tumor invades more than one subsite of supraglottis or glottis, with normal vocal cord mobility.
Glottis (ICD-O topography C32.0):
  T2: Tumor extends to supraglottis and/or subglottis, and/or with impaired vocal cord mobility.
Subglottis (ICD-O topography C32.2):
  T2: Tumor extends to vocal cord(s) with normal or impaired mobility.

In areas where more specificity is needed, the basic categories are further divided (e.g., T2a, T2b).

Beyond the three axes of the basic classification (i.e., T, N, and M), every code can be expanded with prefixes and codes of additional classifications.

Prefixes are coded in small letters and may be combined. The following prefixes are available:

Prefixes

- **c** for a stage that has been determined during clinical examination (c is the default when no prefix is given)
- **p** for a stage that has been determined through pathological methods
- **a** for a stage that has been first determined at autopsy
- **m** for multiple primary tumors (the T stage in that case is defined by the extension of the largest primary tumor)
- **r** for a recurrent tumor, after a disease-free interval, at the primary site
- **y** for a condition subsequent to multimodal therapy.

These additional classifications are provided:

Additional classifications

The *certainty factor* C indicates diagnostic **validity** according to the diagnostic methods employed. Available codes range from C1 (evidence from standard diagnostic means, e.g., palpation, standard radiography) to C5 (evidence from autopsy).

Histopathologic grading G serves to further specify the primary tumor, ranging from G1 (well differentiated) to G4 (anaplastic = undifferentiated).

The classification of *residual tumors* R indicates if part of the tumor remained after surgery. The classes are R0: tumor removed completely; R1: microscopic residual tumor (resection edges); R2: macroscopic residual tumor or unresectable metastases.

Using the classifications L and V, *lymphatic and venous invasion* can be described. There are the classes LX/VX: not assessable; L0/V0: no invasion; L1: lymphatics invasion; V1: microscopic vein invasion; and V2: macroscopic vein invasion.

The usage of prefixes and additional classifications is optional. However, to give a complete picture of the patient's disease stage, all information that is supported by the facts of the case should be given.

These are two coding examples, showing the descriptive power of the TNM system:

Examples

Carcinoma of the larynx:
ICD-O topography C32.0, TNM pT1a pN2b M0 G2 R0 C4
    This code classifies a histopathologically established carcinoma
(pT) of the glottis (C32.0), with moderatedly differentiated histology (G2), restricted to one vocal cord with normal mobility (T1a).
Multiple ispilateral lymph nodes are affected, none of them
greater than 6 cm in dimension (N2b); this fact has also been
histopathologically established (pN). No distant metastases
were detected (M0) when specialized diagnostic procedures
(e.g., imaging procedures) had been applied (C2). After resection (C4), no residual tumor remained (R0).

Carcinoma of the breast:
ICD-O topography C50.4, TNM cT4aC2 N3C2 M1C2
    The code describes a carcinoma that has been assessed pre-
operatively (cT) and that is located in the outer upper quadrant
of the mamma (C50.4) and directly extends to the chest wall
(T4a). Metastases were detected in the ispilateral lymph node
along the arteria mammaria interna (N3) and more distantly,
e.g., in the bones (M1). All these observations are based on
specialized diagnostic procedures (C2), e.g., tumor extension
and lymph node affection are based on a CT scan and bone
metastases on a skeleton scintigraphy.

Note that, because of the different meanings of the same code for
different locations, a TNM code can be understood only in combination with the ICD-O topographical code of the primary tumor.

3.6 MeSH and UMLS

When the U.S. National Library of Medicine (NLM) developed the
Medical Subject Headings (MeSH), the goal was not to code
features of the patient, or of the clinical care process, but to code
the content of medical literature articles. Skillfully applied, the
MeSH nomenclature, which is based on a **polyhierarchical concept system**, can substantially increase the recall and precision of
literature retrieval.

The **Unified Medical Language System** (UMLS), another NLM
product, brings together clinical codes with literature codes in a
so-called meta-**thesaurus**, to establish an automated link between
the clinical case and the pertinent literature.

3.6   Exercises

Exercise 1

What are the primary purposes of disease classifications, medical
procedure classifications, medical nomenclatures, and tumor staging systems?

How many axes does the ICD-10 have? How many semantic di-   **Exercise 2**
mensions underlie its structure?

What are the advantages and disadvantages of the ICD-10-PCS as   **Exercise 3**
a multiaxial, general classification of medical procedures, as compared to the ICPM?

In SNOMED RT, diseases can be described as a combination of   **Exercise 4**
concepts from the dimensions topography, morphology, and etiology (see the ovarian cyst example in section 3.3.1). Doesn't this
make the disease concepts (D7-75111 in the same example) redundant and thus unnecessary? Give reasons for your answer.

Typical Medical Documentation   4

In Chapter 5, we will discuss the uses and benefits of **medical documentation** on a general and methodical level. To prepare for that discussion, we introduce in this chapter the medical documentation typically used in health care institutions. We start with a description of the contents and structure of a **patient record**, followed by an introduction to patient record archives. We introduce the clinical **basic data set documentation**, the tumor **documentation**, **medical registers**, documentation for **clinical studies**, documentation in doctor's offices, and documentation maintained for **quality management** purposes. Many of the examples cited are part of a hospital's extensive documentation tasks. Therefore, we will have a look at the role of documentation in **hospital information systems**, too.

Introduction

In this chapter you will learn
- the typical medical documentation,
- how it is structured, and
- how to utilize it.

What will you learn?

The Patient Record   4.1

The patient record is composed of all **data** and **documents** generated or received during the care of a patient at a **health care institution**.
The conventional patient record physically consists of one or more loose-leaf files; in the outpatient setting, index-cards are often used. An **electronic patient record** is stored in the file system of one or more **computers**. Frequently, these two storage forms are combined. In section 7.3, we will discuss the particular features of the electronic patient record.
The patient record is composed of a number of partial documentation elements (patient history documentation, patient findings documentation, summarizing reports, overviews, etc.); all of them have different characteristics and suit different purposes (cf. section 2.3.1). The patient record in most cases constitutes a patient-oriented, only partially standardized, **content documentation**.

Definition

Every patient record includes the following:
- data to reliably identify the patient: a personal identification number, if available; name and date of birth, supplemented, if necessary, by name at birth and current address;

Content

- further **information** about the patient, including marital status, family doctor, health insurance information, etc.;
- information about the patient's history, complaints, and reasons for seeking treatment;
- information about diagnostic examinations, their results, and the diagnoses derived from them;
- description of therapeutic interventions, e.g., medication, operations, physical treatment, etc.;
- documentation of the course of illness, the response to therapy, eventual complications and their treatment;
- information on the success of the therapy, the patient's condition at discharge, and further therapeutic recommendations;
- summary and critical reflections on a particular phase of the care process, usually as part of the discharge summary.

One single record

One of the guiding principles of **clinical documentation** is to bring together all information pertaining to an individual patient (see section 1.3.1). Thus, each patient in a **health care institution** should have only one single patient record. Dividing a patient record into an outpatient and inpatient record or, for example, into a surgical and an anaesthesia record, impedes the access to important information. Due to their exceptional format, however, some special records, e.g., x-ray bags or tissue samples, cannot be avoided. The main record, then, has to contain clear references to these special records. (For this specific information, the main record becomes a **reference documentation**.)

Internal structure

By gathering several treatment phases in one patient record, the record can become quite extensive and complex. To still be able to find information quickly and reliably, it is crucial to structure the record appropriately. One way of doing that is to separate individual inpatient and outpatient contacts, for example, by using dividing sheets. In many institutions, patient records contain several compartments, organized by categories that reflect the institution's specific requirements. Typical categories are discharge summaries, consultation reports, laboratory results, nursing reports, etc. Within these *source-oriented* categories, the order is usually chronological, with the most recent documents being filed on top.

A lot of work has been done to find a way of replacing the source orientation of the record's structure with a more content-related orientation, e.g., in the *problem-oriented record*. None of these approaches, however, could be demonstrated to actually improve **patient care**. Furthermore, there seems to be an insurmountable tendency in practice to file documents on top of the record in the order of their arrival.

Nowadays, many documents in the conventional patient record are computer printouts, e.g., laboratory results, spirometry results, discharge summaries, operation reports typed into a text processing system, etc. The portion of documents created on a computer will further increase. Thus, it seems natural to strive for a patient record that is completely stored on electronic **document carriers**: the electronic patient record. To achieve that, however, all documents created manually (e.g., the results of a physical examination, the patient history, or the temperature chart) have to be transferred, at a certain cost, into an electronic form (the documents can be scanned, for example). Electronic patient records can be accessed faster, they will get lost less often, they can be copied more conveniently, and they need less archiving space. But whether they can be handled as easily and in as many different ways as conventional records, or whether they even are more useful than conventional records, will depend to a large extent on the design of the **application systems** implementing the electronic patient record. You will learn more on this subject in section 7.3.

Electronic patient record

Patient Record Archives

4.2

A major part of all medical experience is stored in the patient record, which is kept in the patient record archives. But records and archives are often treated carelessly.

Size

Bearing in mind that patient records must be stored for up to 30 years, for each patient bed, depending on the medical specialty, between 4 and 8 meters of shelf space have to be planned in the archives. In a hospital with 500 beds, this means 3000 meters of shelf space for 400,000 patient records. In large university hospitals, the stock of patient records sometimes is bigger than the stock of the university library.

In large archives, it makes sense to file patient records by the patient's date of birth and, within a date of birth, by the patient's current surname. The date of birth is almost always known, unchangeable, and highly selective; thus, the record can be found even after a longer period of time. To distribute the records equally over the archive, they should be ordered primarily by month of birth, then by the day, and finally by the year.

Organization

Patient records that are filed in the wrong place are most probably lost forever. To avoid that, records have to be marked using colored tabs or stickers in a way that misplaced records catch the eye immediately.

The *age* of a patient record is **defined** as the period since the last discharge of the patient. (So, unlike most other things, records can grow younger by usage.) Experience shows that the older the record is, the less frequently it is being accessed. Thus, it is often appropriate to store records of a certain age more cheaply in a *secondary archive*. It takes much more time, of course, to retrieve a record from the secondary archive, but, on the other hand, there is no frequent need for that, and more space in the current archive becomes available.

Every patient record archive that places great emphasis on the **completeness** of its stock has to provide a mechanism for *lending control*. In large archives, there is no way to cope without a computer-based *records management system*.

Alternative storage media

Microfilming of patient records, especially for the secondary archive, leads to an enormous saving of space. Often, the complete secondary archive can be fit into one single microfilm cabinet. The microfilms (or microfiches) are put together and managed just like file cards.

Instead of microfilming, the patient record can be stored on the *optical disk* of a computer (similar to an audio CD). For that purpose, all documents have to be available in electronic form (see document carrier); in most cases this means that at least some documents will have to be scanned first. To ensure permanence of the records (for up to 30 years!) as well as to exclude subsequent changes to them, the writing process on the medium must be irreversible (using WORM devices: "Write once—read many").

The advantages of optical disk archiving increase with the portion of documents that have been created on computers and are available in electronic form.

4.3   Clinical Basic Data Set Documentation

Definition

The clinical basic data set documentation is a **standardized documentation** of a relatively small set of data (typically diagnoses and costly procedures together with some basic characteristics) of all patients of a health care institution. It enables immediate access to records of patients with particular diagnoses, therapies, or other specific **attributes**. Moreover, basic statistics on the structure of the patient clientele of the institution can be performed.

Motivation

The motivation for clinical basic data set documentation in health care institutions includes:
- Legal requirements increasingly demand the compilation and transfer of performance data for all patients of the institution.

- Developments in the funding mechanisms of health care institutions require transparency of the "business" (or treatment)
  processes.
- The mix of patient characteristics and care activities is an indispensable input for business planning.
- The attributes of the basic data set enable the reliable identification of cases for scientific studies based on patient records.

Content

Every basic data set documentation contains some organizational
core elements like the patient's unique identification attributes
(social security number, name, birth date) and details of the contact (time, length of stay, attending physician, mode of discharge,
etc.).
Looking more closely at diagnoses, you can distinguish admission
diagnoses, transfer diagnoses, discharge diagnoses, and epicritical
diagnoses. Each type reflects a different stage of the care process.
The admission diagnosis usually is expected to justify subsequent
diagnostic measures; the epicritical diagnosis is "the last word" on
the case, justifying everything that has been done or not done during the care process.
To reliably and completely retrieve patients with particular diagnoses or therapies, as well as to count and compare the number of
cases, those attributes are **coded** using medical **coding systems**.

MBDS

In Europe, standardized attributes for the basic data set documentation of outpatient and inpatient patient care have been suggested
in the so-called **Minimum Basic Data Sets** (MBDS).

Clinical Findings Documentation

4.4

Content

Unlike clinical basic data set documentation, **clinical findings
documentation** contains the details of many, if not all, findings
that have been produced for a patient during a specific episode of
care. These include laboratory results, results of physical examinations, x-ray results, ECG results, etc. Clinical findings documentation is an essential part of every patient record.

Structures

The clinical findings of a patient may be presented on a large
number of different documents. Their structure may range from
strongly structured documents (like tabulated laboratory results) to
more or less unstructured text (e.g., in radiology result reports).
Due to the large number and diversity of document types it is virtually impossible to standardize the clinical findings documentation for all patients of an institution. When a particular evaluation
requires clinical findings to be **recorded** in a standardized way, a
medical register must be set up that implements **vertical docu-**

mentation for a small **study sample** and enables **prolective analysis** (see section 6.2.3).

Progress documentation

An essential attribute of each clinical finding is at what point in the **course of an illness** or of the health care process it was produced. The *chronological relation* of a patient's findings provides additional information for the health care process. In **progress documentation**, the temporal course of an illness and of the care process are **captured**.

Quantitative parameters (see **level of measurement**) that have been measured repeatedly over time can be presented graphically in a *progress chart*. Examples are the fever chart, the glucose level chart of the glucose tolerance test, and the blood pressure chart during operations. Among the first design considerations for a new progress chart are the adequate frequency and duration of the attribute's observation.

If the results are of a qualitative nature (see level of measurement), or if graphical presentation is not required, *progress tables* may be used. The values of several attributes, represented in the rows of the table, are given for different points in time, represented in the columns. Cumulative laboratory reports are typical progress tables. The simplest form of progress documentation are *progress notes*, a continually updated document with more or less structured, date-stamped (sometimes time-stamped) textual notes.

4.5 Clinical Tumor Documentation

Motivation

The demand for documentation during the course of the treatment of a tumor is particularly high for several reasons:

- The approach to diagnosis and therapy is highly interdisciplinary. In many cases, the specialty for the affected organ (e.g., gynecology) is supported by other specialties, especially surgery (for tumor resection), internal medicine (for chemotherapy), and radiology (for staging and radiation therapy).
- Treatment extends, in general, over a long period of time, and its desirable and adverse effects must be continuously balanced.
- Tumor aftercare requires close diagnostic monitoring to identify recurrent tumors and metastases over time.
- Clinical research depends on detailed data from long-term, patient-oriented observations.

Tasks

Clinical tumor documentation primarily serves **patient-oriented analyses**. Its most important tasks are to support the coordination and organization of all diagnostic, therapeutic, and aftercare activities. For that purpose, selected data of all treatment episodes are collected from outpatient clinics, hospitals, and doctors' offices to serve as a basis for further decisions. These data may also be useful to provide organizational support like patient visit scheduling and automatic processing of appointment reminders.

Moreover, tumor documentation provides the central information resource for cancer epidemiology. In many cases, systems for tumor documentation have direct **communication links** to regional or national **cancer registers**.

Content

In the context of oncological patient care, tumor documentation constitutes basic data set documentation. For selected patients, it can be expanded by additional attributes to allow more specific analyses, often for research purposes. Essential attributes of every tumor documentation are the time of the first tumor diagnosis; information about the type of the tumor, its localization, histology, and oncological stage (e.g., the **TNM system**; see section 3.4); important therapeutic interventions; and, possibly, the time of death. Since various tumor diseases show quite different characteristics and courses, specific variations of documentation have to be planned.

Organization

Data acquisition takes place at the health care institution, usually performed by the treating physician. The set of data, standardized to a large extent, is then transferred to the regional oncological center or any other institution coordinating the patient's care on the regional or even national level.

Duplicate data acquisition for the purpose of tumor documentation could be avoided by **logical data integration** with the health care institution's **information system**. The overlap of the need for data both in tumor documentation and in current hospital information systems is so small, however, that more reliable patient identification and better control of completeness might be the only advantages of **data integration**.

Documentation for Quality Management

4.6

Motivation

In many countries, there is a legal obligation for every health care professional to secure an appropriate **quality of patient care**. For health care institutions, it is an economic necessity to make every effort to assure (and manage) the quality of their services (see quality management).

Three aspects of quality

Often, quality of patient care is described from three viewpoints: the quality of a health care institution's structure, the **quality of the care process**, and the quality of the treatment results (**outcome quality**). The quality of an institution's *structure* refers to the facilities, the technical equipment, and the staff's level of training and knowledge. The quality of the care *process* describes the degree of correspondence between the actual health care activities and the accepted principles of clinical practice. To achieve high quality of the care process, you might make sure, for example, that a tumor patient is always being seen and assessed by representatives of all relevant medical specialties (e.g., an internist, a surgeon, and a radiotherapist). Outcome quality, finally, is an assessment of the treatment results. Leaving financial aspects aside, it is basically the success of a treatment—measured by the duration and quality of the patient's ongoing life—that determines the quality of the care process. These long-term criteria for the success of a treatment are very difficult to measure and even more difficult to attribute to a certain **health care intervention**. This is why, in practice, quality of patient care is often assessed by judging the appropriateness of the care process by accepted standards or as compared to other health care institutions.

The role of documentation

Medical documentation contributes to the quality of the care process. It may supply valuable information for evaluating the quality of the care process as well as outcome quality. On the one hand, it provides the basis for case reviews, i.e., a comprehensive retrospective evaluation of individual courses of illness. On the other hand, there might be a prospective and continuous observation of selected **quality indicators** for a predefined set of treatment cases, to assess the general quality standards, for example, of all heart surgeries in a region. This is called **quality monitoring**.

Quality indicators

Quality indicators have to be selected carefully. They have to be reliably observed and with adequate costs, and they must be sufficiently valid measures of the relevant quality aspect. Quality indicators are, for example, the consumption of certain drugs (like antibiotics or psychoactive drugs), the frequency of complications (e.g., after surgery), and the success rates of certain therapies. Serious methodical and organizational problems arise in the observation and interpretation of long-term success criteria like survival rates, changes in the quality of life, and remission rates. Attributes of the patient's satisfaction with the care process should be part of every quality assessment.

External obligations

Aside from activities of internal quality management, the health care system usually imposes obligations on health care institutions to report quality measures for external assessment. To enforce these obligations, they are frequently connected to accreditation or reimbursement processes.

Clinical and Epidemiological Registers

4.7

Generally speaking, every standardized documentation of health care data for a predefined study sample of treatment cases, striving for completeness within this sample, may be termed a medical register. A medical register serves the systematic **patient-group analysis** of the data, usually to answer clinical or epidemiological research questions.

In a **clinical register**, the study sample is restricted to the clientele of one or a few health care institutions. Great caution has to be used, therefore, in applying the findings of clinical register analyses to other parts of the population. Typically, analysis is guarded by questions on specific factors influencing the success of a therapy or, more generally, the patient's prognosis (like age, gender, or particular findings), as well as on the **incidence** of complications or other undesirable events within the health care institution.

Epidemiological registers try to cover a certain region (e.g., a state) as completely as possible with their study sample. Most of the epidemiological registers serve the research into serious and not too frequent diseases (there are, for example, cystic fibrosis registers, cancer registers, echinococcosis registers, etc.). A typical analysis investigates the incidence or **prevalence** of a disease in the region of interest, stratified by differential diagnoses, gender, age-group, etc., and tries to identify an increasing number of cases (e.g., of leukemia near nuclear installations) as well as decreasing numbers (e.g., after vaccination programs).

There is an important point to keep in mind when analyzing a medical register: In contrast to experimental clinical studies, the data reflect the observation of courses of illness, which usually do not permit any causal conclusions. When analyzing an epidemiological register you may find, for example, that the proportion of smokers among patients with high blood pressure is higher than among the overall population. But this doesn't prove that smoking is a cause of hypertension. Maybe the typical smoker shows some characteristics that distinguish him or her from the rest of the population and that can be responsible for hypertension as well (e.g., stress at work or lack of exercise). So again, the interpretation of results requires great caution. If the register has not been planned and implemented carefully, a whole range of different biases may render the results of an analysis completely unusable.

Organizational support

Apart from estimators for the prevalence and incidence of diseases, medical registers can also provide valuable planning data for clinical and epidemiological studies, possibly dealing with questions that were raised only in the analysis of the register data. Moreover, registers may also support organizational tasks as they come up, for example, in the aftercare of chronically diseased. There are registers with highly specific organizational tasks, for example, transplantation registers or optimizing the **allocation** of available transplants in large areas.

4.8 Documentation in Clinical Studies

Clinical studies

Clinical studies are meant to answer two types of questions:
- How useful is a particular diagnostic procedure?
- How effective is a certain therapy for a given indication, and is it equivalent to, or even better than, the established (standard) therapy?

Every clinical study follows a study plan that establishes in detail the time points for examination, the examination procedures, statistical methods, etc. For data acquisition, specific *case report forms* are developed to produce a well-structured and standardized **data record** (see standardized documentation). Apart from the study's end points, which are of primary interest, there are concomitant diseases, supportive medication, and undesired events that have to be recorded and **classified**.

The role of documentation

Studies that are intended to support the registration of a new drug, as well as scientifically ambitious studies, must apply particularly high standards for data quality. Each single data item must be verified carefully, and its correctness must be made credible (data monitoring). Data of doubtful correctness are presented to the treating physician for correction in a *data query*. The process of data correction is also part of the documentation. Finally, the data are released for **statistical analysis**. All study documents are archived in the *trial master file*.

Regulations and guidelines

The process of planning, conducting, and analyzing clinical studies is subject to the legal regulations of the countries in which they are carried out, or in which the new drug is to be registered. Many of these regulations refer to international guidelines, especially those gathered in the **good clinical practice** (GCP) guidelines. For every important activity involved in the execution of a clinical study, **standard operating procedures** (SOPs) have been formulated in these guidelines.

In Chapter 8, we will describe the details of **data management** in clinical studies.

See Chapter 8

Documentation in Hospital Information Systems   4.9

A hospital information system is the partial system of a hospital which stores, processes, and exchanges information. It consists of information procedures and all human and technical agents in their role as information processors.

The fundamental objective of a hospital information system is the provision of information about patients and their care, about the quality of patient care, about performance and expenses of the health care institution, as well as the provision of **medical knowledge**.

Hospital information systems

Documentation is of crucial importance in hospital information systems. All information provided by a hospital information system, has to be collected, **indexed**, ordered, and stored. That is, it has to be documented. All data management systems described in this chapter may be part of a hospital information system.

The role of documentation

Due to its importance and complexity, documentation in hospital information systems is described in detail in Chapter 7.

See Chapter 7

Exercises   4.10

What information should a patient record contain? Which types of analyses should be possible?

Exercise 1

Which additional ways of analysis does an electronic patient record offer compared to a conventional record?

Exercise 2

What are quality indicators? What characteristics should they have?

Exercise 3

What conditions have to be met so that the analysis results of medical registers can be generalized to other parts of the population.

Exercise 4

Exercise 5   There is no exercise 5 in this chapter.

Exercise 6   What is the benefit of tumor documentation whose data accurately
reflect the current state of the treatment
-   to the patient?
-   to the treating physician?
-   to medical science?

Utilization of Clinical Data Management Systems   5

In section 1.1 we emphasized that the point of **medical documentation** is not to collect **information** but to utilize collected information in a sensible way.

In this chapter we describe problems that often arise when using **data management systems**, and we introduce methods that can help to solve them.

The chapter has three sections referring to three different categories of use, each of them presenting typical problems and requiring typical methods: patient-oriented (or casuistic) analysis, patient-group reporting, and analysis for **clinical studies**. Even if we introduce a method as being typical for one specific category, this is not to say that it cannot be applied beneficially in the other categories.

In this chapter you will learn
- the fundamental tasks associated with **patient-oriented analyses**, patient-group reporting, and analyses for clinical studies;
- how to recognize problems that typically arise with these tasks;
- methods that can help you to respond to these problems in a systematic way.

Patient-Oriented Analysis   5.1

A patient-oriented (or casuistic) analysis of medical documentation focuses on the determination of information about a single identifiable patient. This information is mainly needed to manage the patient's health care process in a well-informed way. This includes the selection of the next steps in diagnosis and treatment as well as continuous control during their application. The latest laboratory results, for example, seen in connection with all previous information about the patient, can prompt a diagnosis and a treatment order, or the suspension of the current treatment, or at least an order for additional diagnostic tests. Moreover, the **documentation** can provide the basis for a sound prognosis about the future course of the patient's illness, e.g., within the context of a medical expert report.

On the other hand, the patient-oriented analysis of documentation can be helpful for the critical review of health care actions:

- In **quality management**, especially within the context of postgraduate or continuous training of health care professionals, documentation can provide indications of the appropriateness of the measures taken and the skillfulness of their implementation.
- In legal proceedings, documentation is quoted to prove or disprove treatment errors.

In scientific research, **anonymized** descriptions of individual treatment cases serve the presentation of particularly typical or particularly atypical courses of illness.

Problems and requirements

Problems with patient-oriented analyses usually arise when important requirements are not met:
- Information about a patient is difficult to find, or is incomplete, unless there is an unambiguous and permanent reference of every piece of **data** to the patient. A surname can change, the date of birth can be keyed in incorrectly, and the combination of both—even if they are correct—is not necessarily unique to a single person.
- Relevant information is missing either if it has not been **recorded** or if it is stored at a place where it cannot be accessed. Due to the highly specialized medicine of today, information about one patient is usually distributed over many different locations.
- Once accessed, information about a patient cannot be used efficiently if it is presented in a confusing way, or if it is just too extensive: Usually only part of the information available about a patient is relevant for a specific task.
- Regulations to ensure data confidentiality and **professional secrecy** typically restrict the permission to analyze documentation in a patient-oriented way. In any data management system, technical and organizational precautions have to be taken in order to prevent unauthorized patient-oriented analyses as far as possible.

Important methods

There are a number of methods available that can help to make a data management system satisfy the above-mentioned demands. The most important methods include the following:
- **Surrogate keys** can support the correctness of the patient reference. Using surrogate keys, often supplemented by centrally stored **demographic patient data**, the **referential integrity** of distributed data can be controlled systematically. Patient identifiers that are calculated from the date of birth and the last name of the patient, have proved not to be useful due to their variability in time.

- Use **standardized documentation** to increase **completeness**. In some situations, this can simply be achieved by prescribing the structure of a history sheet, as follows: (1) patient identification and demographic data, (2) current disease history, (3) history of former diseases, (4) family history, (5) social background.
- Methods of **data integration** will enable you to gather distributed information about an individual patient from several departments of a **health care institution** or from several health care institutions. Current laboratory findings can be passed on automatically from the laboratory to the requesting ward via a **communication link**.
- For the **computer**-based presentation of information to the health care professional, a number of methods have been proposed (see Chapter 4). Generally speaking, the goals are
  - to underline similarities through a uniform presentation,
  - to highlight differences and exceptions,
  - to present information in a structured way but without structures that distract the reader's attention,
  - to facilitate orientation by using screen-representations of well-known paper forms and other real-world **objects** like notepads, file-card boxes, or dictating machines (so-called metaphors).

Summary

In patient-oriented analysis, health care–related information about an identifiable patient is sought in order to manage the health care process in a well-informed way. Documentation serves as a memory aid and a means for **communication** between all the caregivers involved. Retrospective reviews of the care process usually rely on patient-oriented analyses of the documentation. To be able to fulfill these tasks, documentation has to be complete, and every piece of data must be accessible, comprehensible, and unambiguously connected to a single patient. Confidentiality and professional secrecy must be ensured.

Classification

Looking back at our typology of clinical data management systems in section 2.3, we can say that patient-oriented analysis requires data management systems that
- contain primarily clinical facts (**class** C1) and
- allow patient-oriented analyses (U1 or U3).
None of the other features are predetermined by patient-oriented use.

Examples

Patient-oriented analyses in many cases rely strongly on **documents**. Most of these have standardized and well-known structures, so that they promote clarity of the presented information.

Some typical documents for patient-oriented analyses are (cf. Chapter 4) history sheets, clinical examination reports, result reports (laboratory, x-ray, etc.), nursing care charts, operation reports, progress charts, and discharge summaries.

Checklist: Patient-Oriented Analysis

Task

Provide health care–related information about identifiable patients to those who are entitled to see it.

Objectives

The main objectives of patient-oriented analyses are
- the management (including the planning and control) of a patient's health care process,
- the prognosis of the future course of the patient's illness,
- the critical review of health care actions taken (or not taken),
- the presentation of prototypical (or very atypical) cases to the scientific community.

Problems

Problems in patient-oriented analysis can arise due to
- data with an ambiguous reference to the patient,
- incomplete data or data that are distributed over several locations in an uncoordinated way,
- insufficient clarity of data presentation.

Methods

Customary methods include
- the use of surrogate keys for the identification of **data objects**, together with other mechanisms to ensure referential integrity;
- the standardization of documentation;
- mechanisms for **logical data integration**, e.g., procedures of systematic communication between **application systems**.

5.2 Patient-Group Reporting

Tasks of the documentation

Patient-group reporting supplies aggregated information about a predefined group of patients (or about all patients) of a health care institution. This aggregated information consists, for example, of the frequency of certain events or conditions (complications, diagnoses, etc.), or of measures describing **quantitative attributes** (e.g., the duration of a treatment in terms of the mean, the standard deviation, or the quantiles). There are several tasks that require patient-group reporting:
- Rules and regulations for the reimbursement of services or for the accreditation of health care institutions may demand regular reports to health insurance companies or to accreditation or-

ganizations, containing measures like the frequency of diagnoses, therapies, or complications, the average duration of treatments, etc.

- To be able to plan and control the work processes of a health care institution, the management board needs highly detailed information about the costs accrued for the treatment of particular groups of patients (**defined** by a common diagnosis or treatment procedure).
- Within the context of quality management, patient-group reporting can be implemented to continually monitor **quality indicators** in patient groups receiving particular **health care interventions** (e.g., **quality monitoring** of complication rates in patients receiving total hip replacements).

In patient-group reporting, certain requirements have to be met in order to avoid inaccurate results and false interpretations:

Problems and requirements

- To obtain valid patient-group information, there is a need for standardized documentation under comparable conditions, i.e., a need for **observational equivalence**. For example, the frequency of a diagnosis in different patient groups can be compared only if the diagnosis was made according to standardized criteria and **classified** using a common **classification** with identical rules.
- Incomplete **data acquisition** can have adverse consequences: interventions that have not been recorded will not be paid for; treatment expenses may be judged inappropriately by the payer if the documentation fails to report serious findings, complications, relevant comorbidity, etc.
- Although patient-group reports are intended only to describe observations of a defined scope, their results tend to be generalized beyond this scope. These generalizations will be flawed by the above-mentioned deficiencies as well as by ill-structured, incomplete, and ambiguous reports.
- Usually, health care professionals are badly motivated to **capture** data for patient-group reporting. Few of them know the harmful consequences that inadequate data acquisition can have; in many cases, they are not even aware of the purpose of a particular report to which they are supposed to contribute information.

The implementation of patient-group reporting requires systematic planning, including the following steps:

Important methods

- Design the layout for a clear and unambiguous presentation of results and specify it, e.g., in sample result sheets.

- From this design, derive the **attributes** that have to be captured in a standardized form in order to achieve these results, as well as their **value sets**.
- Check whether the necessary attributes have already been captured in another context (and probably with better motivation to obtain quality data) and therefore can be re-used for this purpose. Discharge summaries might contain, for example, high-quality diagnoses that can be used for morbitity reporting, or for case-mix analyses.
- Develop organizational precautions and rules to guarantee completeness and **reliability** of documentation. Physicians, for example, may be required to encode the discharge diagnoses of their patients after sufficient training in the use of the classification.
- Choose adequate computer-based tools to support the process of data acquisition, data integration, and reporting.

Summary

To allow patient-group reporting, a data management system has to provide aggregated information about defined groups of patients. This information is required in order to comply with external rules and regulations, to be able to plan and control the work processes of an institution, and to support quality management. Valid reports must be based on complete and reliable data, obtained under comparable conditions. To be useful, reports have to be unambiguous and well structured. Today's demands on the complexity of patient-group reports as well as the need for data integration usually call for the use of computer-based tools.

Classification

Looking at our typology of clinical data management systems in section 2.3, **patient-group analysis** can be said to require data management systems that
- contain clinical facts (class C1 or C4),
- allow patient-group analyses (U2 or U3),
- are at least partly standardized (S2 to S4),
- at least contain some horizontal elements (D2 or D3),
- contain directly documented elements (R2 or R3),
- are supported by **computer systems** (T1 or T2).

Examples

These are typical examples of patient-group reports (some of them already mentioned in Chapter 4): regular reports on the frequency of diagnoses, case groups and operations for a hospital's inpatients, used for case-mix analyses, statistical reporting, etc.; reports to the hospital's management on the number of patient contacts in an outpatient clinic, the average duration of contacts, the consumption of resources for certain groups of patients, required to analyze cost-benefit structures; quality management reports, indicating waiting times, complication rates, wound healing times, and other quality indicators, required to identify problems and to assess the effect of interventions.

Checklist: Patient-Group Reporting

Provide aggregated information about defined groups of patients (or all patients) of a health care institution, using frequencies and other statistical measures.
Task

Objectives typically include:
Objectives
- to fulfill external rules and regulations, often connected to accreditation and reimbursement;
- to provide information on cost-benefit structures and on the features of the institution's work processes, needed for planning and management;
- to monitor quality indicators of the institution's work processes in order to detect problems early and assess the effect of interventions.

Problems often arise due to
Problems
- differences in the care of patients (in terms of quality or costs) not being reflected by the documentation's data as a result of incomplete data acquisition or of the data's too coarse granularity;
- similarities in the care of patients being obscured by variations in the documentation process, caused, for example, by using different measuring procedures, data capturing forms, or **coding systems**;
- relevant results and implications of the data escaping notice because they are presented in unclear, ambiguous, or unnecessarily detailed reports.

Common methods include
Methods
- standardized documentation,
- systematic planning of the documentation with regard to the kind of results expected,
- increase of completeness by **multiple use of data** and organizational precautions.

5.3 Clinical Studies

Tasks of the documentation

In preparation and support of clinical studies, **medical data management systems** may be expected to provide the following functions:

- To support patient selection according to defined attributes (e.g., all male patients over the age of 60 and suffering from bladder carcinoma. The selected patients then form the **study sample** of a separately planned clinical study.
- To provide information useful for the planning of such a clinical study, for example, on the variability of potential end point **variables**, on potential confounding factors, and on the structure of the study sample.
- To provide new medical insights by generalizing the observations made in a set of patients in a defined scope. For example, the data might be analyzed to find patient characteristics that influence the outcome of a certain therapy. This kind of generalization requires statistical methods.

To be able to answer the last kind of question, the data management system either has to have documentation of a clinical study, or has to take the form of a **medical register**. Let us have a short look at these two important **concepts** of clinical research.

Medical registers

Medical registers are medical data management systems with an emphasis on scientific medical research. Over a longer period of time (usually without a defined termination date), patients of one or more health care institutions are included into the register following explicit inclusion criteria. The set of attributes captured for each of the patients has been defined with certain research questions in mind, but may be expanded in the course of time as new questions arise. Medical registers are analyzed periodically in order to demonstrate temporal trends.

Interventional studies

In comparison, clinical studies extend over a limited period of time and have a defined termination date. They deal with the examination of precise and usually strictly limited research questions. In a narrow sense, clinical studies are *interventional studies*, where therapeutic or diagnostic interventions are varied systematically (e.g., by randomized **allocation**, see below). Interventional studies are also called **clinical trials**. In Chapter 8, we describe the documentation of interventional studies (especially **therapeutic trials**) in more detail.

Observational studies

In a broader sense, clinical studies also comprise observational studies, where the course of treatment of patients in a hospital or a doctor's practice is observed, documented, and analyzed—interfering with the treatment process itself as little as possible. In the **retrospective study**, patients who have experienced a specific target event (e.g., a disease or a complication) are selected. The study then sets out to establish factors that might have caused or favored that event. For comparison, a group of patients is chosen who have not (yet) experienced the event (the control group). This kind of study is called a *case-control study*. There is an option to examine and question the patients about possible influencing factors after selecting them for the study (thus ensuring that all necessary examinations are been taken and questions are been asked). It is more convenient, however, to just analyze the records of the selected patients. This makes the study retrolective, i.e., the study sample is defined after the time of data acquisition (see section 6.2.3). The trade-off for convenience here is that actual influencing factors might be overlooked because nobody had thought of asking that particular question at the time of the patient contact.

In a **prospective study**, patients or persons sharing a specific characteristic (e.g., showing a certain risk factor, receiving a particular treatment) form the study group, whereas the control group consists of persons lacking this characteristic. Both groups are observed in order to spot certain target events (e.g., the appearance of a disease, a complication, or the death of the patient) that might be a consequence of the patient characteristic in question. This is called a *cohort study*. It can be carried out retrolectively, i.e., exclusively on the basis of treatment reports. To achieve reliable results, however, observations and their documentation should be made with the goals of the study in mind, i.e., the study should provide a prolective design.

If the analysis of a medical register or a clinical study is to yield correct and complete results that can be reliably interpreted, a number of requirements have to be fulfilled:

Problems and requirements

- The attributes of all observed data objects have to be recorded in a standardized way. However, even standardized documentation can produce invalid results when observational equivalence is not guaranteed.
- Comparative studies with two or more groups of patients can only be interpreted when **structural equivalence** between these groups exists. This turns out to be a considerable restriction since an entry in a medical register is usually not preceded by randomized allocation of health care interventions.
- If results of an observed patient group are intended to be generalized to a **target population**, the study sample has to be representative of that population.

- **Validity** of the attributes is of major importance: Do the captured **attribute values** really reflect the patient characteristics that matter?
- Generally speaking, any reliable scientific study must be planned, carried out, and analyzed systematically right from the beginning. Further investigation of this aspect is the subject of medical biometry.

Important methods

The success of any scientific clinical study depends on the use of appropriate methods. Basically, the following aspects have to be considered:

- The precise formulation of the questions of interest must be the starting point for the establishment of the attributes and value sets forming a standardized documentation. This ensures reliability of the data and comparability of data objects.
- Attributes should be chosen to be objectively observable in order to achieve observational equivalence; otherwise, additional methods are required to ensure comparability.
- Structural equivalence between compared groups can be achieved reliably only when the members of the groups are assigned by **randomization**. To a certain degree, matching procedures or stratified analysis can be applied instead, e.g., in medical registers.
- Only a careful definition of the study sample and the target population in the planning phase of a study guarantees the study is representative. The evidence of studies based on medical registers is often restricted to a target population consisting of future patients of the health care institutions contributing to the register. As a guideline for the systematic planning of medical registers and controlled clinical trials, generic study plans (so-called protocols) have been suggested. When complying with them, the interpretability of the results will improve considerably.

Summary

In support of clinical studies, a data management system or a medical register is supposed to allow the selection of patients for a study according to defined attributes; to provide information useful for the planning of a study; or to be the information basis of a study, enabling new scientific insights by analyzing the documented observations. For all these tasks, observational equivalence between all of the patients in the documentation must be ensured. The attributes used in the analysis must be a valid equivalent of the patient characteristic in question. If groups or patients are to be compared in order to detect the effects of certain interventions or conditions, the groups must be structurally equivalent.

In trying to classify data management systems that support clinical studies according to our typology in section 2.3, we can say that they

- will contain clinical facts (class C1 or C4),
- must enable patient-group analyses (U2 or U3),
- must include standardized elements (S2 to S4),
- will have in-depth (vertical) elements (D1 or D3),
- must contain directly documented elements (R2 or R3),
- will have at least some computer support (T1 or T2).

Here are some types of questions of interest that would typically be posed to medical registers (there are others that we already mentioned in section 4.7):

- How frequently does a given condition (a disease, a risk factor, etc.) or a certain event (the onset of an illness, the occurrence of a complication, etc.) arise in a defined patient group?
- What is the distribution of certain quantitative attributes (see **level of measurement**) in a defined patient group? (What is the average systolic blood pressure? To what degree does the white blood cell count vary in a healthy population?)
- What influences do certain attributes have on the patient's prognosis or his or her response to a certain therapy?

Examples

Checklist: Clinical Studies

To prepare and support scientific clinical studies with information determined by patient-group analyses.

Task

The objectives of patient-group analyses for clinical studies are

- to select patients with certain characteristics for a specific study,
- to plan a study efficiently on the basis of previous observations,
- to analyze documentation with regard to concrete questions of interest.

Objectives

Analyses produce biased or incorrect results in cases of

- poor observational equivalence between cases,
- poor structural equivalence between patient groups, or,
- poor **representativity** of the observed patients for the target population.

Problems

The most important methods include

- systematic planning of all aspects of the study from the formulation of the questions to the methods of analysis (set down in

Methods

the study protocol and continuously monitored during the implementation of the study);

- randomized allocation of interventions in experimental studies, substituted, if necessary, by matching;
- standardized methods for treatment and documentation.

5.4 Quality Measures in Information Retrieval

Precision and Recall

The point of any documentation is to allow the retrieval of information stored in it. Thus, the quality of documentation to a large extent depends on whether information can be retrieved completely and specifically. To express this quality, the measures of **precision** and **recall** have been introduced.

Let us assume that a user phrases a query to a data management system that stores a set D of data objects (e.g., treatment cases). Let us further assume that a subset R of set D is relevant for the user's question (the set R is exactly what the user would like to retrieve). As the actual result of the query, however, the system delivers (selects) a set S of objects (or cases).

These sets are illustrated in Fig. 5.1.

relevant		**selected**		
		Yes	no	total
	yes	$R \cap S$	loss	R
	no	noise		
	total	S		D

Fig. 5.1 Contingency table to illustrate the different sets of data objects pertaining to precision and recall in information retrieval.
D: set of data objects in the database;
R: set of data objects relevant to the user's question;
S: set of data objects selected by the query (the result set).

The measure of precision describes the proportion of the selected objects that are relevant for the user's question. It can be calculated as $|R \cap S| / |S|$ ($|X|$ denoting the number of elements of a set X). The measure of recall, on the other hand, describes the proportion of relevant objects that were selected by the query. It can be calculated as $|R \cap S| / |R|$.

Recall and precision are opponents, or antagonists. One is often increased at the expense of the other.

Exercises   5.5

When carrying out scientific clinical studies, observational equivalence is of major importance. How can it be achieved?

Exercise 1

Besides observational equivalence, in some scientific clinical studies, structural equivalence is a crucial point. What kind of studies are these and how can structural equivalence be achieved?

Exercise 2

How would you characterize a medical register?

Exercise 3

In documentation that serves patient-oriented analysis, it is usually appropriate to acquire information in a nonstandardized way. Give reasons why elements of standardized documentation might be sensible even for a purely patient-oriented analysis.

Exercise 4

For your documentation of hospitals, what kind of utilization would you imagine (refer to Chapter 2, exercise 5)? How do you take into account the corresponding requirements and methods?

Exercise 5

Why is it much more difficult to determine a query's recall than its precision in practice?

Exercise 6

Clinical Data Management: Let's Make a Plan!   6

Medical **coding systems** and **medical data management systems** can be very complex constructions. Whether they achieve the objectives they aspire to depends on the appropriate selection and the proper use of the available methods and schemes.

Developed intuitively, without a deliberate plan, such systems carry the risk of putting a considerable burden on everybody involved—without producing satisfactory results.

In this chapter you will learn
- why medical data management systems and medical coding systems have to be planned systematically;
- important design principles for medical coding systems;
- how to evaluate existing coding systems and to construct simple coding systems of your own;
- the principles of systematically planning medical data management systems and an exemplary scheme for its implementation.

Planning Medical Coding Systems   6.1

General Principles   6.1.1

When you plan a new medical coding system, you should first clarify whether you will need a **classification** or a **nomenclature**, i.e., whether you want to *categorize* or *describe* facts in the first place. Additionally, and independent of this choice, you should heed the following principles:
- Keep to a single **semantic dimension**. If one dimension isn't enough for your purpose, design a **multidimensional classification** or nomenclature. The dimensions then have to be independent of one another.
- Select the **concepts** and their **authorized terms** in accordance with the **documentation** task at hand.
- All concepts have to be **defined** and circumscribed clearly.

In a classification you have to be careful that
- the selected **classes** cover the semantic dimension completely (to be on the safe side, you add the class "Others" on all hierarchical levels), and

- the classes are mutually exclusive. If necessary, you have to establish rules to make the assignment of an **object** to a class reliable (Table 6.1).

Table 6.1 Example for intersecting class contents (cf. the disease chapters of the ICD).

Code	Preferred term
c1	Infectious diseases
c2	Malformations
[...]	
c6	Circulatory diseases
c7	Respiratory diseases
[...]	

Where would a bacterial pneumonia fit in? And a malformation of the heart? The contents of the classes overlap due to diverging semantic dimensions (etiology, morphology, and topography).

Using the following classification rule, a reliable assignment can be safeguarded:

c7	Respiratory diseases
	excluding: Infectious respiratory diseases ($\rightarrow$ c1)

It is obvious that an extensive classification without a uniform semantic dimension (e.g., the ICD) needs a large number of classification rules (which do not exactly make its application easier). To limit the number of rules, a set of general rules is formulated like, for example, that the localization always has priority over the pathological process (or vice versa).

6.1.2   Principles of Ordering Qualitative Data

Well-defined concepts

Principle 1: In contrast to classifications, a nomenclature does not require its concepts to be mutually exclusive. Nevertheless, their contents should be clearly circumscribed (Table 6.2).

Use hierarchies

Principle 2: When designing a coding system, you should always consider the use of a **hierarchical concept system** as its basis. If there are clear hierarchical relations between the concepts you use, they should be represented in the coding system. The concept hierarchy enables a top-down design of the coding system; when used in encoding later on, it will make the retrieval of authorized terms much easier. Moreover, in a **hierarchical coding system** the intended meaning of each concept is made more explicit by fitting it between superordinate and subordinate concepts. In that way, **terminological control** of documentation is enforced; it is exactly the **consistent** ordering of the concepts, however, that makes the creation of a coding system so difficult.

Table 6.2 Example risk factors: mutually nonexclusive concepts in a nomenclature.

Code	Preferred term
i1	no risk factor
i2	adiposity
i3	arterial hypertension
i4	nicotine abuse
i5	alcohol abuse

As opposed to classifying, indexing does not force you to select exactly one code within each semantic dimension. An overweight person who chain-smokes can be described by the tuple (i2, i4).

To make the application of concepts reproducible, one might define, e.g., arterial hypertension as a systolic value greater than 21.3 kPa and/or a diastolic value greater than 12.6 kPa.

The entry "i1: no risk factor" of the nomenclature is a special case: it excludes all other entries. This might be fixed in an indexing rule: "i1: no risk factor; excludes i2 to i5." One might also erase i1 from the nomenclature, concluding that there is no risk factor if no one is indicated. But then the implicit meaning of i1, that "risk factors were sought for, possibly even more than those mentioned in the nomenclature, but none were found", will be lost.

Principles of Ordering Quantitative Data

6.1.3

For most tasks, quantitative **data** can be used directly (see **level of measurement**). For others, they are ordered by size and ranked. Every time that observations must be counted and tabulated, quantitative data have to be **classified**. There has to be a projection, accordingly, from the numeric **value range** of the **attribute** into a classification. The classes of the classification are the result of splitting up the value range into intervals. The following principles apply:

Why order them?

Principle 1: The intervals have to cover the value range completely and must not overlap (Table 6.3).

Exhaustive and mutually exclusive intervals

Principle 2: In most cases it is appropriate to divide the value range into intervals of the same length (Table 6.3). The class limits are then equidistant.

Equidistant class limits

Principle 3: To avoid many sparsely filled classes at the end of the scale, you may introduce "open" classes, e.g., "≥70 years of age" (Table 6.3).

Open classes at the end of the scale

Table 6.3 Example: Exhaustiveness, mutual exclusiveness, and equidistant class limits in classifying quantitative data.

wrong Notation	Class description	right Notation	Class description
<10	younger than 10 years	≤ 9	0 up to 9 (full) years
10-20	10 up to 20 years	10-19	10 up to 19 years
20-25	20 up to 25 years	20-29	20 up to 29 years
25-30	25 up to 30 years	[...]	
30-40	30 up to 40 years	60-69	60 up to 69 years
40-70	40 up to 70 years	≥ 70	70 years or more
>70	older than 70 years	n. s.	age not stated

The classes of this classification overlap. The variable class width might be justified in a situation where most patients are between 20 and 30 years of age and where differences between 20- to 25-years-old patients and 26- to 30-years-old patients are of particular interest.	The last class is necessary to fulfill the condition of exhaustiveness. It must be made clear that full years are the basis of calculation and that even a day before his or her 20th birthday, a person still belongs to the class 10-19.

6.2 Planning Clinical Data Management Systems

6.2.1 Why Plan Them at All?

The knowledge of the specific objectives ...

In Chapter 1 we depicted the possible objectives of **medical documentation**. Each **data management system**, implemented in a practical setting, pursues only a portion of these objectives and introduces its own specific subobjectives. Additionally, there is always a range of general and specific side conditions—be they legal, organizational, staff-related, or financial—to be taken into account.

...ensures sufficient but minimal effort

In developing or improving a data management system, you should be careful to meet exactly those requirements that result from the specific objectives and side conditions. Each additional effort would be wasted, and each effort falling short of the requirements could endanger the success of the whole system.

Systematic planning

Thus, planning a data management system requires, as a first step, the detailed analysis of objectives and side conditions so that, in a second step, the requirements on the system can be derived and justified.

For the sake of completeness, **reliability**, and accountability, this process should follow explicit guidelines. In our view, the use of explicit guidelines is the key characteristic of the **systematic planning of data management systems**.

The Documentation Protocol

The **documentation protocol** provides an explicit guideline, or scheme, for the systematic derivation of system requirements from the documentation's objectives. Thus, it constitutes a method for the systematic planning of data management systems. The "study protocol," a long-proven method in planning and conducting **clinical studies**, serves as a model for the documentation protocol.

Table 6.4 provides a proposal for the structure of a documentation protocol. It demonstrates four major sections:
- the formulation of specific documentation objectives, motivated by concrete problems to be solved;
- description of the future system's tasks, resulting from the specific objectives;
- derivation of the system design, based on the complete set of tasks;
- description of organizational and technical side conditions for the development, introduction, and use of a data management system.

In section 6.3 you will find a simplified example of a real documentation protocol.

Table 6.4 The documentation protocol: proposed structure.

0 Introduction
0.1 The documenting institution
0.2 Participants
0.3 Motivation for the project
	3 Conceptual design of the data management system
	3.1 Data storage
	    3.1.1 Conceptual design of the documentation scheme
	    3.1.2 Catalogue of attributes
	3.2 Data acquisition
	    3.2.1 Organization of the acquisition process
	    3.2.2 Design of data acquisition forms
	3.3 Computer-based communication
	3.4 Security concept
	    3.4.1 Data privacy
	    3.4.2 Data and program security

1 Objectives of the documentation
1.1 Problems and objectives
1.2 Evaluation of the starting-point
    1.2.1 Current state of knowledge
    1.2.2 Possibilities and limits of the current system	

2 Specification of documentation tasks
2.1 Questions and tasks
2.2 Definition of evaluation samples
2.3 Methods for analysis
    2.3.1 Standardized recording methods
    2.3.2 Biometrical methods
2.4 Result presentation layout
	4 Side conditions
	4.1 Project organization
	4.2 Documentation tools
	
	5 Modifications to the last protocol version

6.2.3 Prolective and Prospective Analyses

The situation

At any moment during the planning or running of a data management system, the wish may arise to use it for answering a certain question or fulfilling a specific task. The next step then is to think about which **data objects** have to be **captured** and to which outside-world objects they belong, i.e., the **study sample** is defined.

Prolective: question first

At this point, we have to make a distinction: If the study sample is defined *before* even part of the data has been captured, the process will result in a **prolective analysis** of the documentation (analysis with preselection): The objects are selected (and the data-**object classes** are defined) before **data acquisition** takes place.

Retrolective: data first

Otherwise, the analysis will be retrolective: The data are captured before the objects are selected (analysis with postselection). In a prolective analysis, data acquisition can be adapted to the specific questions, whereas in a **retrolective analysis**, you will have to work with the data already captured. In many cases, this makes a considerable difference in the quality of the results!

Prospective: looking forward

Do not confuse, however, prolective with prospective! In **prospective studies** (studies looking forward), possible effects (e.g., diseases) of given factors (e.g., exposure to a risk) are investigated. For example, workers vulcanizing rubber (exposure to a potential risk) are observed with regard to future diseases they might develop.

Retrospective: looking backward

Accordingly, studies looking for the possible cause of an observed effect are called retrospective. Adapting the example above, patients with chronic bronchitis would be asked whether they ever worked in a rubber factory.

6.2.4 Additional Remarks

Effects of poor planning

As we have already explained, poor planning of medical data management systems can lead to an implementation that does not meet its objectives. But even if the objectives are met, poor planning can cause unnecessarily high expenses. This occurs, for example, when the **multiple use of data** is not ensured and the same data have to be captured more than once, or when the operation of the system is not in line with the work processes of the employees. For example, **information** that emerges in the patient's room has to be jotted down on paper intermediately if the **computer** for **data entry** is located in the ward office.

These—and more—efficiency issues have to be recognized in the planning phase of a data management system, because at this time the most efficient countermeasures can be introduced. Here we have one more important benefit of the systematic planning of data management systems.

Example: A Tumor Documentation Protocol   6.3

Here is an example of a tumor data management system (see section 4.5) that was planned systematically according to the structure proposed in Table 6.4. Note that documentation protocols can differ considerably depending on their specific objectives and side conditions. We give only a shortened version of the protocol's contents because of space limitations.

All names and data used in the example are fictitious. The example's contents, however, are based on a real documentation protocol.

Documentation Protocol for an Area-Wide Basic Tumor Data Set Documentation of the Marbletown/Ploetzberg Tumor Center (MPTC)

1st version, passed by the steering committee of the common tumor center of the Marbletown University Hospital and the Ploetzberg General Hospital and Medical School on November 11, 2000.

0 Introduction

0.1 The Documenting Institution

Contractual partners of the MPTC are the Marbletown University Hospital and the Ploetzberg General Hospital and Medical School (PMC), termed "participating hospitals" in the following passages.

All patient care units of the participating hospitals are obliged to capture basic tumor data for all their oncological patients and to transfer these data to the tumor center.

0. 2 Participants

Participants in the basic tumor data set documentation are:
- the participating hospitals as documenting institutions,
- the Department of Medical Informatics of the PMC in the capacity of gathering, storing, and analyzing the data,
- the steering committee of the tumor center, serving as a decision-making body and as a consultant to the Department of Medical Informatics.

0. 3 Subject and Motivation

Malignant tumor diseases are the second most frequent cause of death in Germany, after circulatory diseases. Due to the severe course of these diseases, there are extensive demands on documentation to support diagnosis, therapy, and aftercare, as well as to answer questions in current research.

The MPTC has been founded to optimize the care of cancer patients in the Marbletown/Ploetzberg area. A regionally complete documentation, crossing the borders of single institutions, is a prerequisite for the effective work of a tumor center. A computer-based data management system is to be developed ("TuDoc"), which meets the requirements of basic tumor data set documentation.

1 Objectives of the Documentation

1. 1 Problems and Objectives

An important task of the tumor center is to contribute to high quality of patient care and to tumor research in a region. To be able to assess and to improve aspects, the steering committee needs a current overview of all oncological patients being treated in the participating hospitals. In the same way, the leading physicians of the participating hospitals should be able to monitor patient care in their institution in terms of medical quality and of treatment costs. Finally, researchers in oncology need detailed and reliable data. The data available at present in the participating hospitals are not suitable for these requirements.

The basic tumor data set documentation has the following objectives:

Objective 1: Current overview of all tumor patients treated and cared for in the participating hospitals

Objective 2: Support of the patient care process

Objective 3: Support of medical research

1.2 Starting Point, Present Data Management System

In the participating hospitals, part of the data necessary for the basic tumor data set documentation are already being stored in computer-based application systems on a routine basis. Since these data differ in the various documenting institutions, they cannot be pooled easily. Moreover, the attributes needed for the basic tumor data set documentation are not being recorded completely. There is an intention, however, to link all available data to the TuDoc system via communication interfaces.

2 Specification of Documentation Tasks

2.1 Questions and Tasks

2.1.1 (Selection) Questions referring to objective 1: Current overview of all tumor patients treated and cared for in the participating hospitals

Q1.1 What is the annual incidence rate of primary tumors in the MPTC and in the participating hospitals?

Q1.2 How many patients have been treated and documented in the MPTC and in the participating hospitals in a specific year?

Q1.3 For how many patients does the documentation cite the date of death?

2.1.2 (Selection) Task referring to objective 2: Support of the patient care process

The TuDoc system has to manage appointments for aftercare. A reminder function for appointments has to be implemented in the scheduling system as well as a function to generate written appointment request to patients.

2.1.3 (Selection) Questions referring to objective 3: Support of medical research

The basic tumor data set documentation serves to answer the following research questions:

Q3.1 How is the frequency of different cancer types distributed along the tumor localization?

Q3.2 What is the frequency of one, two, or more primary tumors occurring in one patient?

Q3.3 For how many patients have relapses been observed?

Q3.4 Has the survival rate of patients with mamma carcinoma in stage X increased over the last decade?

2.2 Evaluation Samples

The evaluation sample is composed of all tumor patients with malignant tumors (ICD-9 classes from 140 to 208 or ICD-10 classes C00 to C97, "malignant neoplasms") who are being treated or cared for in the participating hospitals. Only patients with a con-
firmed diagnosis of malignant tumor disease are admitted to the evaluation sample.

2.3 Analyses

Standardized Recording Methods

Diagnoses are encoded using the four-digit codes of the ICD-10 as well as the ICD-O. Staging information of malignant tumor diseases is encoded additionally, using the TNM system.

Calendar dates are recorded in the format dd/mm/yyyy. All other attributes are provided, as far as possible, with value sets to be chosen from.
At certain points, it has to be possible to enter free-text commentaries.

Regular Reporting

The Department of Medical Informatics of the PMC carries out analyses at regular intervals to answer the questions Q1.1–3 and Q3.1 for each individual clinic as well as for all clinics together. An annual report, containing analyses aggregated over all participating clinics, is sent to the management board as well as to the heads of all departments and institutes. In addition, the heads of all clinics receive an annual report with analyses pertaining to their clinics. The period covered by the report is one calendar year; the report has to be presented in the second quarter of the following year. If required (e.g., when a problem in the quality of patient care is suspected), additional quarterly reports for individual clinics can be ordered.

2.4 Presentation Layout

Under this heading of the documentation protocol, a layout for the presentation of analysis results has to be designed that considers all information needed to answer the questions put in section 2.1. For that purpose, two essential aspects have to be considered:

– What kind of information has to be presented?
– How is it to be presented?

Here, we will give a short example for the presentation layout on the basis of question 3.2. The numbers in Fig. 6.1 are necessarily fictitious; they serve as an illustration of the presentation layout.

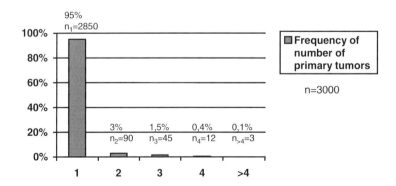

Marbletown/Ploetzberg Tumor Center
Annual report 2000

Fig. 6.1 Design of the presentation layout to answer question Q3.2 on the frequency of different numbers of primary tumors in individual patients.

3 Data Management System

3.1 Data Storage

3.1.1 Conceptual design of the **documentation** scheme

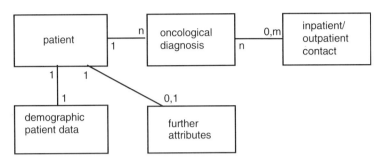

Fig. 6.2   Design of (a part of) the documentation scheme of TuDoc.
One or several oncological diagnoses can be assigned to one patient. There will
be none, one, or several inpatient or outpatient contacts to treat one or more of
the patient's oncological diagnoses. A patient's demographic data are acquired
and are usually supplemented by further attributes.

3.1.2 Catalogue of Attributes

General personal attributes of a patient	name, address, date of birth, gender, unambiguous patient identification code
Further attributes for answering question Q1.1	oncological diagnosis (free text), oncological diagnosis (ICD-O), tumor staging information (TNM system), date of primary diagnosis, primary diagnosis made at a participating hospital of the tumor center
Further attributes for answering question Q1.2	admission date, discharge date, attending hospital, intention of contact (diagnostics, therapy, aftercare)
Further attributes for answering question Q1.3	Has the patient died? If yes, date of death. Is the cause of death related to the tumor?
Further attributes for fulfilling the task referring to objective 2	start of therapy, end of therapy, dates for aftercare
No further attributes are needed for answering questions Q3.1 and Q3.2	
Further attributes for answering question Q3.3	Did a relapse occur? If yes, date of the relapse diagnosis

3. 2 Data Acquisition

3.2.1 Organization of the Acquisition Process

All data are acquired from the patient records and recorded by medical record assistants of the participating hospitals. All data describing a patient and his or her hospital stay are to be recorded as early as possible. After an inpatient stay, data acquisition should reasonably take place immediately after writing the discharge summary.

A list of the doctors and assistants responsible for documentation is attached (Attachment 1). To ensure the completeness of the tumor documentation, all admission and discharge diagnoses recorded in the central patient database are checked for correspondence with the inclusion criteria of the evaluation sample. In case of correspondence, the patient data are transferred to the tumor center. Attachment 2 contains the form for the patient's consent to this data transfer.

3.2.2 Design of Data Acquisition Forms

In this section of the documentation protocol, the screen layout for data entry into the computer-based application system TuDoc is designed in detail, based on the considerations made in sections 3.1.1 and 3.1.2. Since all participating hospitals are sufficiently equipped with modern computer systems and are connected to the hospital's local area network, there is no need to design paper-based forms for data recording.

3.3 Computer-Based Communication

Demographic patient data are transferred from the central patient database via a standardized communication interface to TuDoc, using the technical means of a communication server. This makes duplicate data entry unnecessary. As soon as a patient's data are entered into the hospital's TuDoc application system, they are transferred immediately to the central TuDoc application system in the tumor center. The communication server is used for this purpose, too. The central TuDoc application system returns a receipt to the local TuDoc system.

3.4 Security Concept

3.4.1 Data Privacy

The Department of Medical Informatics of the PCM takes care that the data are protected against unauthorized access and that data are transferred only with the owner's consent. The owner is responsible for the compliance to all data privacy and confidentiality regulations.

The following arrangements are made:
- restricted data access (differentiated access privileges for persons working in different roles and in different clinics);
- anonymized analyses, as long as they are not exclusively directed at the head of a hospital or clinic;
- personalized analyses for individual patients are restricted to the analyzing clinic's own data.

3.4.2 Data and Program Security

The Department of Medical Informatics of the PCM stores all TuDoc applications and data on the tumor center's central computer on behalf of the participating hospitals. There is a daily backup for all data.

3.5 Legal Requirements

Storage and processing of data take place in accordance with German legal regulations. Reporting to the regional epidemiological cancer register is done in accordance with the Regional Epidemiological Cancer Registry Act. The annual report of anonymized tumor data to the central tumor register of the German Association of Tumor Centers conforms to common law.

4 Side Conditions

4.1 Project Organization

Data acquisition takes place in the participating hospitals.

The Department of Medical Informatics of the PCM is responsible for the provision, service, and maintenance of the TuDoc software, which is used for data entry and storage of the basic tumor data set documentation. All functions are developed and implemented in coordination with the participating clinics. The medical informatics department also ensures data quality (e.g., integrity and plausibility checks).

4.2 Documentation Tools

To support basic tumor data set documentation, the computer-based data management system TuDoc will be introduced. TuDoc presents screens for data entry and offers functions for patient data management, for the transfer of data to the Department of Medical Informatics of the PCM, and for the printout of the data records. Data recorded with TuDoc are encrypted and stored redundantly on the hard disk of a local computer so that a clinic can analyze its data in its own application systems. The Department of Medical Informatics consults the clinics on how to design and implement such analyses.

System requirements for the local TuDoc application systems: XYZ operating system, at least xx MB of RAM and at least xx GB of hard disk space; ABC-network adapter; color printer.

5 Documentation Period

From January 1, 2000, until further notice, all participating hospitals will carry out the basic tumor data set documentation in accordance with this version of the documentation protocol.

6 Signatures

Head of the MPTC's steering committee
Medical Director of the University Hospital Marbletown
Medical Director of the Ploetzberg Medical Center

Protocol attachment 1:   Doctors and documentation assistants responsible for the basic tumor data set documentation
Protocol attachment 2:   Form to record the patient's consent to reporting data to the tumor center.

6.4   Exercises

Exercise 1   At which points does the structure of the documentation protocol in section 6.3 differ from the proposal in Table 6.4? Think about possible reasons.

Exercise 2   Design the result presentation layout for the questions referring to objective 1 of the documentation protocol in section 6.3.

Exercises 3-4   There are no exercises 3 and 4.

Exercise 5   Referring to exercise 5 in section 5.5, develop the documentation protocol for your hospital documentation. Alter former decisions, if necessary. From now on, you should plan all documentation with regard to the analyses you want to carry out, i.e., prolectively. The planning process should be recorded in a documentation protocol.

Documentation in Hospital Information Systems   7

Hospital information systems are among the most important and most complex **information systems** in health care. A hospital without **clinical documentation** is scarcely conceivable.
This is why you will never find a hospital information system without elements of clinical documentation.
The **electronic patient record** is of growing importance for any **computer**-supported hospital information system.

In this chapter you will learn
- the importance and the extent of hospital information systems;
- about the close connection with medical (and especially clinical) **documentation**;
- about the benefit and the problems of electronic patient records and strategies for their introduction.

The Hospital Information System   7.1

The Concept   7.1.1

What is a hospital information system? In the literature you will find many different **definitions** and various views on hospital information systems. To begin with, we see a hospital information system as a subsystem of the hospital that processes and stores **information**. Much of the information stored and processed is an element of **medical documentation** that becomes, in turn, an integrated component of the hospital information system.
Even if **computer systems** and networks (the hardware) and the **application systems** installed on them (the software) are of particular importance, there is more at stake than that: the processing of **data**, information, and **medical knowledge** in the hospital as a whole.

The **concepts** of **information and knowledge logistics** were introduced in Chapter 1. A hospital information system is supposed to provide
- information of all kinds, especially about patients;
- medical knowledge, especially about diseases, but also about **health care interventions**, e.g., the desired and undesired effects of drugs and the interactions between them;

- information about the **quality of patient care** and about the performance and costs of a hospital.

In university hospitals, there are additional tasks in teaching and in research. Also, we should not forget all the working areas we listed in section 2.1.2 relevant to hospital information systems.

According to the definition in section 2.2.3, medical knowledge is a particular kind of information. Hence, when we talk about information in the following sections, we are including medical knowledge.

7.1.2 The Significance

Quality factor

The information system of a hospital is a quality factor. Virtually all groups of people working in a hospital need enormous amounts of information for their activities. The better these needs can be met, the higher the quality of care as well as of the hospital's management.

For example, for a newly admitted patient, the first thing a physician needs to know is the reason for admission and the most recent medical history. Later, the results of diagnostic tests are supplemented. Eventually, he or she might also need pieces of the most current medical knowledge, concerning differential diagnostics or therapeutic methods for the diseases in question. If this information arrives too late, or is obsolete, or even wrong, this will affect the quality of care. A time-consuming search for information as well as redundant examinations may become necessary, which will increase the costs of **patient care**.

There is a natural demand **to record** information in a way that it can be used by other persons involved in the care process: documentation as a **communication** aid (cf. section 1.3.2)!

The administrative staff in the hospital has compelling information needs as well. Missing or inaccurate information may cause a failure to charge for all services that were performed, and reduce the income of the hospital. Money will be lost when information comes in too slowly and reimbursement is delayed for days or even weeks—money that could be better spent on patient care.

The management board of a hospital needs information about the performance and costs of the hospital as well as about the volume and the quality of patient care. The spectrum of diseases treated by a department and the complication rate of a certain surgical procedure are just two examples of that type of information.

The information system of a hospital is a considerable *cost factor* as well. We assume that about 3% to 5% of the costs of an enterprise are connected with computer-based information processing. Those cost estimations comprise investment costs as well as operation costs (including staff). Considering the information system as a whole, the proportional costs are even higher: Some analyses calculated the proportion of information processing costs in hospitals to be about 25%. This is a considerable amount of money, bearing in mind that, for example, in 1996 in the European Union (EU), the costs for health care, including the costs for 14,000 hospitals, amounted to 814 billion Euro; which is 8.7% of the total gross domestic product (GDP) of all EU countries. Looking at these numbers, you will easily imagine the potential cost savings that may be brought about by efficient information processing.

Cost factor

Information processing in hospitals can and should convey an integrated view of the patient and the hospital. In that way, some of the undesirable side effects of highly specialized health care processes can be avoided. Information about an individual patient can be brought together and presented clearly, even if the data are acquired by many different persons in various departments of the hospital. It is not only the physician treating a patient (cf. **casuistic analysis**) who gains from integration, or the management board aggregating data from several departments in cross-patient analyses; it is virtually every person working in the hospital.

Integrated view

In a figurative sense, an information system can be regarded as the *memory and the nervous system* of a hospital. It receives information to process it, transmit it, and store it in order to make it available when needed. Whether the system hospital is able to recognize relevant facts, to remember them, and to act accordingly—all this depends to a considerable extent on the quality of information processing.

A metaphor

The Need for a Strategic Plan

7.1.3

The need for a strategic information management plan of a hospital's information system arises from the mere fact that almost all groups of persons and all areas in a hospital are affected and may profit from a high-quality information system.

Range of users

It is also the volume of information being processed in a hospital every day (and night) that strongly demands a strategic plan of the information system. A typical university hospital, for example in Germany, is an enterprise with about 5000 employees, an annual

Volume of information

budget of about 350 million Euro, and a multitude of tasks in re-search, teaching, and patient care. About 50,000 inpatients and 200,000 outpatients per year trigger the production of approximately 20,000 operation reports, 250,000 discharge summaries, 20,000 pathology reports, 100,000 microbiology reports, 200,000 radiology reports, and 800,000 clinical chemistry reports. Every year, about 300,000 new **patient records** with about 7 million pages are created. Archiving them in the conventional way, this makes up about 1500 meters of records per year. Patient records usually have to be kept up to 30 years, at least in Germany. In digital archives, the data volume is estimated to be 5 terabytes per year.

There are conventional and computer-based tools available for information processing. Looking at a university hospital today, the computer-based tools usually comprise a two-figure number of large, interoperating application systems, a four-figure number of workstations (or PCs) and other terminal devices, as well as a two- to three-figure number of large computer systems, usually linked by a high-speed network.

Multiple usability of data

It is sensible to do all of the information processing of a hospital in an integrated way. The most important reason for this is that the information needs of the various groups often refer to the same data. A careful strategic plan of a hospital information system is necessary to achieve multiple usability of these data (see section 1.4). Duplicate **data acquisition** and **data analysis** lead to unnecessary costs of information processing.

Integrated information processing is advantageous not only to the patients and the staff of a hospital, but also to health insurance companies and to the owners of a hospital. All information barriers put up between professional groups or departments will generate redundancies, inconsistencies, unnecessary costs, and inferior patient care.

Systematic information processing

The above discussion emphasizes the importance of a systematic approach to a hospital's information processing. This pertains also to medical documentation, as a part of the hospital information system (cf. section 6.2). Investments in information processing tools have to be made according to a strategic plan. There must be clear agreements on all processes and the responsibilities involved, and the interfaces between all the components must be described carefully.

Important Hospital Functions

Introduction

In this section we introduce the important functions in a hospital that process information and thus form a part of its information system. Since information needs are continually growing, just as information technology is continually progressing, there will always be additional functions.

Patient data management

When a patient arrives at the hospital, he or she is first admitted administratively. At this point, the **demographic patient data** are recorded and unambiguous identification **codes** for the patient and the hospital visit are issued. In addition, it is important to know whether there is any information about the patient from earlier visits. In that case, the identification codes and the demographic patient data must be transmitted to those responsible for the treatment along with the patient record created at the earlier visit.

To record demographic patient data and make them available, a patient **data management system** has to be implemented. It forms the kernel of a hospital information system's memory, because all clinical information must relate to a uniquely identified patient. To meet these requirements, a number of software products are on the market, that usually also support reimbursement procedures as well as management functions on the wards and in outpatient departments.

Ward management

On the wards, the hospital information system has to support health care professionals in their duties. There are many administrative tasks, such as the admission and discharge of patients, and the ordering of services (e.g., laboratory and x-ray examinations, but also food, drugs, and materials). Documentation activities are of particular importance: the documentation of diagnoses and interventions (examinations, therapies, nursing activities) as well as their results and any other relevant information gained during the patient's health care process. All this information forms part of the patient record where paper-based **documents** still play an important role. There are software products, however, that support a number of management functions, like ordering meals, drugs, and materials; ordering patient records at the record archive; and providing online access to important documents like discharge summaries, operation reports, and diagnostic result reports. The purpose of all tools, conventional as well as computer-based, is to minimize the time and materials spent by an improved organization. Duplicate diagnostic tests are avoided, the documentation process is simplified, materials are procured faster and easier, and the local stocks are reduced.

Management of outpatient clinics

There is considerable overlap of the tasks on the wards and the tasks in outpatient clinics. In the outpatient clinics, the hospital information system can be of some help in making appointment scheduling more efficient and supporting the control of work processes. Since the turnover of patients is significantly higher in outpatient clinics than in wards, quick and easy access to the patient record or individual documents is of crucial importance here.

Documentation of surgical operations

Much time is spent in planning and documenting operations. Information about operations is of particular importance, however, for the care process (operation report) as well as for the administration (services to charge, resource consumption, overall costs of an operation, etc.). **Computer-based application systems** can make a valuable contribution to planning and documenting operations, and they may facilitate the writing of the operation report.

Diagnostic service units

Diagnostic service units of a hospital, like clinical chemistry or radiology, produce a huge amount of diagnostic reports every day. The hospital information system can help control the work processes, which are usually very well structured. The production and storage of result reports, as well as their transmission and presentation, is a natural domain of the information system in diagnostic service units.

Among the most important requirements are reliable **communication links** with the application systems of the requesting departments and the hospital management. This will not work if there is no hospital-wide, unambiguous identification of the patient and of the relevant unit of reimbursement, or "billing case." Pursuing the idea of multiple usability of data, the record of the services performed should emerge as a by-product for the hospital management. There are specialized software products on the market for most of the different types of diagnostic service units.

Patient record archives

The stock of a hospital's patient record archive is extensive and sensitive, and requires adequate protection (cf. sections 4.1 and 4.2). This is why efficient information processing can be of particular value. An important task is the management of every record from when it is started until it is old enough to go into long-term secondary archives, including close lending control in the meantime.

The efficiency of the management and the access to the record improves considerably when all documents of an individual patient are filed in one integrated record.

Thus, a computer-based application system for records management should be closely coupled to the central patient database. The electronic patient record (cf. section 7.3) offers complete integration, along with the utilization potentials that result from it.

Administrative functions make sure that all external services of the hospital are reimbursed. Moreover, administrative functions comprise financial management, accounting, investments, and costing, as well as the management of human resources, facilities, and materials.
All these functions need data from wards, outpatient clinics and service units—from wherever direct or indirect health care services are provided.
For administrative functions, standard software products are available on the market, as these functions are required in every enterprise, not only in hospitals.

A great number of medical reports are dictated or drafted by physicians every day and subsequently transformed by typists into typescripts or computer files. There are, for example, discharge summaries, operation reports, and diagnostic result reports. The almost ubiquitous availability of computer-based text processing tools has facilitated the creation and correction of reports considerably. Above that, a hospital information system has to provide means of cooperatively drawing up reports, and of storing and presenting them in a patient-related way. A good reporting system lets medical reports be produced in time, stored safely, retrieved quickly and reliably, and presented adequately.
Moreover, a hospital information system needs functions for the cooperative writing of documents and for the patient-referred management and presentation of them, in order to draw up the documents in a timely fashion, to retrieve them reliably, and to present them in a suitable manner.

The clinical **basic data set documentation** is an important component of a hospital information system. Since it contains data on all patients in the hospital, the sheer volume of the data absolutely requires computer-based tools. The functionality to record, store, and analyze the basic data sets is integrated in many of the software products for patient data management (see above).

It is one of the most important tasks of the hospital management to plan and control the central work processes in the hospital. An integrated hospital information system increases transparency of these process by providing information about which services were provided for what kinds of patients at which units of the hospital. There are specialized software products available on the market;

they can only be used efficiently, however, if sufficient **data integration** has been attained.

Quality management

Information processing plays a crucial role in a hospital's **quality management**. The hospital information system is expected to provide relevant data about the work processes, about the patients and their illnesses, and about diagnostic and aspired therapeutic standards (cf. section 4.6). Hence, **multiple use of data**, information, and medical knowledge is indispensable for the efficient management of the quality of patient care.

Access to medical knowledge

Due to the huge and ever-growing volume of medical knowledge, it is necessary for doctors, nurses, and all other health care or administrative professionals, to access **bibliographic database systems** and knowledge bases right from their workplace (examples: bibliographic database systems like **MEDLINE**, clinical practice guidelines, knowledge bases for diagnostic and therapeutic decision support).

7.1.5 Exercises

Exercise 1

Compare the tasks of a hospital information system with the objectives of medical documentation. Do you find that they overlap, and, if so, what are your conclusions?

Exercise 2

Draw the connection between the hospital functions introduced and medical documentation.

7.2 Management and Operation of Hospital Information Systems

Introduction

The exemplary functions of a hospital information system that we described above have to be carefully planned and adequately designed, and their operation must be continually monitored. These are tasks of the management of hospital information systems, which are often carried out in the form of projects. Examples of such projects might be the introduction of a new application system for clinical chemistry, or a study to check the timely transmission of diagnostic result reports.

Strategic decisions that concern the hospital information system as a whole regularly have to be made. Due to the high costs and the profound organizational effects, there is strong demand for long-term planning. Setting up a high performance computer network in a hospital with several buildings and thousands of rooms is not a half-year project.

There are two important prerequisites for the systematic management of a hospital's information processing: the availability of highly skilled, specialized staff; and the clear **allocation** of responsibility and authority for decisions concerning staff or investments. Before a software product is selected and purchased, or before it is developed in-house, a requirements analysis is usually done, which leads into an invitation to tender. After the purchase, the software product must be adapted to the requirements of the institution and installed (it must be customized). The introduction of the application system must be preceded by adequate usage training of the staff involved.

At several points in this chapter it has become clear how decisive the multiple use of data (cf. section 1.4) is for the efficiency of a hospital information system. But this is only possible if all information about a patient arising anywhere in the hospital is brought together correctly (see **referential integrity**) and is made available to the professionals involved in the care process. To do so, every data item must be tagged with an unambiguous identification (a **surrogate key**) of the patient and the case. Organizational aids like adhesive **labels** or magnetic cards must carry the same identification tags that are used in the computer-based application systems.

Due to the multitude of functions, like the ones we described in the previous section, large hospitals often use several application systems implemented on several computer systems. Those application systems cannot be regarded independently but must be able to cooperate ("interoperability"): they either share a common database or they exchange **messages** via a communication system. Sometimes it makes sense to keep the same data redundantly in various application systems. In this case, the **consistency** of redundant data must be carefully ensured: as soon as data are added, changed, or deleted in one application system, the same modification must be triggered in all other application systems (see data integration, referential integrity).

Every effort should be made to support the work processes on the wards and in outpatients clinics by a single application system, the health care professional workstation. This system should be easy and fast to use, and it should be shared by physicians, nurses, and other health care professionals. It should provide all functions needed by these professional groups, but not every function will necessarily be accessible by members of every group.

All aspects of the privacy of patients and employees, and the necessary protection of data, have to be considered in the management and operation of a hospital information system.

7.2.1 The Strategic Plan

Design guidelines

A strategic plan will be useful for the long-term planning of a hospital information system, as it sets general guidelines for the design process. The following statements could be taken from the strategic plan of an existing hospital information system.

Examples

- Within the next five years, a set of common functions will be introduced to support quality management in the hospital; the functions will draw, among others, on regular standardized reporting.
- The current laboratory information systems are obsolete and are too expensive to maintain. To replace them, a suitable software product has to be selected, customized, and implemented.
- If possible, only application systems should be introduced that provide standardized communication interfaces and disclose their database structures. This serves for the improved interoperability of the systems.
- To keep service costs small, the number of operating systems and of database systems should be kept as low as possible. Ideally, only one operating system and one database system are used.

7.3 The Electronic Patient Record

Introduction

The electronic patient record and its relevance to patient care have been discussed on a national and international scope for quite some time. In following these discussions you will notice that there are diverging ideas about what an electronic patient record actually is, or should be.

In this section, we introduce our point of view; it is oriented strongly toward the documentary objectives that apply to the electronic record just as they do to the conventional record. Once more, this highlights the close connection between medical documentation and hospital information systems: On the one hand, the electronic patient record is a natural and important part of the hospital information system, whose architecture has a crucial influence on its quality. On the other hand, the methods of planning, designing, and exploiting data management systems, as introduced in this book, retain their full **validity** for the electronic patient record.

What Is an Electronic Patient Record?

To be able to define the electronic patient record, we start by recalling that a patient record is composed of all data and documents generated or received during the care of a patient at a **health care institution** (see section 4.1). Every patient record is characterized by the expression of (at least) the following **attribute types**:

- Data or **document carrier**: The carrier may be conventional (e.g., a sheet of paper, an x-ray film) or electronic (e.g., a hard disk, a CD). The data are stored on this carrier either permanently (e.g., on paper, microfilm, or on CD-ROM) or require an additional, permanent storage device (as data stored on a hard disk or notes jotted on a blackboard).
- **Completeness**: If a particular carrier holds only a portion of all documents, or data, for a patient, it is called a partial patient record. Otherwise we have a complete or comprehensive patient record.
- Availability: At a certain point in time, a patient record can be accessible to only one or to several persons. It can either be accessed only at the place of its physical storage, or may also allow remote access. A considerable time lag may occur between data acquisition and their availability in the patient record. It might take several days, for example, before all current result reports are filed in the conventional record, or before all paper-based external documents are scanned and linked into the electronic record.
- Degree of structuring: In the simplest case, a patient record is just a pile of documents (i.e., letters, forms, notes, result reports, etc.), filed more or less in the order they were produced during the process of care. In search of a particular document, one has to browse the whole record from beginning to end. Since this takes too much time, most of the patient records are internally structured by arranging different types of documents in sections (see section 4.1). Those sections can be adapted in the design of an electronic record. The electronic patient record, however, allows deeper structures: A single patient **attribute** (e.g., the blood pressure) may be stored independently of the document on which it was originally recorded (e.g., the history sheet or a progress note). Later it may be combined with other attributes and presented in various forms, depending on the purpose of the presentation (e.g., in graphical or tabular form, or as a phrase in a discharge summary). To make this

possible, the electronic patient record requires an elaborate internal data model.

Archiving
- Archiving method: After an episode of care at an institution is finishing and documented, the patient record is archived (see section 4.2). Paper-based records are commonly filed in conventional archives, but they might also be microfilmed, or scanned and stored electronically. You would transfer electronic patient records to electronic archives. What you need here is a permanent electronic document carrier, e.g., the CD-ROM. Several partial patient records on different document carriers often prevent integrated archiving and impede later retrieval.

Most of the electronic patient records today are still partial records, supplementing and sometimes repeating the conventional record. In that sense, every computer-based application system for clinical documentation contains a partial electronic record.

The comprehensive approach to the electronic patient record is much more demanding. All data and documents referring to a patient are available completely and exclusively in electronic form, and they are archived on a permanent electronic **storage medium**.

7.3.2 Advantages and Disadvantages of the Electronic Patient Record

Advantages
These are the advantages that are commonly attributed to the electronic patient record:
- The record is available at different places at the same time, usually without any delivery time.
- It is almost impossible to lose.
- Depending on the user (e.g., physicians, nurses, administrative staff) documents and data can be selected differently and presented in different forms; there are different views on the data. The use of views may also benefit data privacy.
- Assuming a sufficient degree of internal structuring (see above), data may be combined and presented in different ways for particular tasks (mean values may be calculated, progress charts drawn, summaries generated, etc.). This promotes the multiple use of data, the deliberate exchange of information, and the efficiency of the documentation as a whole.
- Using specialized views on the patient record, the organization of patient care can be improved, e.g., by listing all examinations that have been ordered, or all missing results.

Disadvantages
Despite of all these advantages, there are also some disadvantages to the electronic patient record. First, it creates a strong depend-

ence on complex technology. There are serious questions, for example, about the record's availability at any time and place that it is needed, and about the staff's ability to handle it with the skills necessary to exploit its potential and achieve reliable results.

Other questions concern the costs: A comprehensive electronic patient record is quite expensive. Its introduction might only be economical if it leads to a complete replacement of the conventional record archives. But this is hampered in many countries by a host of organizational and legal problems.

Introducing the Electronic Patient Record

7.3.3

Early planning

Introducing a comprehensive electronic patient record requires long-term systematic management. If the conventional record is to be replaced, it must be done in a stepwise process. These steps should be set down in the strategic plan (see section 7.2.1). All relevant user groups should be involved in the complete process of planning and implementation in order to achieve their support and acceptance.

Stepwise introduction

The first step of the introduction of an electronic patient record would be to provide carefully selected documents of particular importance in electronic form. These might include textual reports (discharge summaries, operation reports, result reports, etc.), tabular results (e.g., from the laboratory), and medical images (x-ray, CT, MRI, etc.). Frequently, the information contained in clinical basic data set documentation can be exploited to produce a useful overview of a patient's hospital contacts, problems, and health care activities, by way of an index to the patient record.

Hospital-wide access to health care professional workstations

In a more advanced introduction phase, the electronic patient record should be accessible from all areas of a hospital. This requires a pervasive, hospital-wide network with adequate transmission capacity. There must be networked health care professional workstations in all wards, outpatient clinics, doctor's offices, operating theaters, etc. The workstations should provide the functionality of the electronic patient record along with the functions of patient management, drug ordering, access to medical knowledge, etc.

Electronic archives

Despite the growing proportion of electronic documents, the "paperless" hospital today still seems to be a remote ideal. There might be a continuing need for some paper-based documents. To build a completely electronic archive (and thus justify the costs for the electronic record), these documents have to be scanned and coded (i.e., indexed or **classified**). The attributes used to code a document depend to a large extent on the structure and the use of the electronic patient record. At any rate, they must include the patient identification, the date of creation and receipt, the originator, and the type of the document (e.g., external admission for patient by Dr. X., dated 11-01-2001, received 11-03-2001.)

7.4 Methodology of Medical Documentation

Under ideal circumstances, a comprehensive electronic patient record covers the whole clinical documentation of a health care institution. Its success is measured by the degree of fulfillment of a clinical documentation's objectives, as they are formulated in section 1.3. Thus, the successful introduction of an electronic patient record requires not only methods for the management of information systems (see section 7.2) but also methods for the **systematic planning of data management systems** (see section 6.2).

Even if you want to introduce only a partial electronic patient record, you should start by carefully creating a **documentation protocol**. In case you want to use an electronic patient record's potential to present different views of the same data, you first have to identify all different objectives, uses, and side conditions. On that basis, you may design presentation forms (tables, graphs, structured reports, etc.) and a comprehensive data model. To be able to perform analyses requiring **standardized documentation**, you have to provide the attributes with **value sets** that match the principles of a medical **concept system**. Only then will the electronic patient record be more efficient to use and produce more reliable results than a conventional patient record.

A question of particular relevance is how to design an electronic patient record so that it may support the health care process of a patient across the borders of a single institution, or even of a single country, regardless of differences in organization, reimbursement, or language. The question is how to get away from the institution-centered case records and create electronic records that are truly patient-centered.

Data Management in Clinical Studies   8

In section 5.3, we introduced **clinical registers** and **clinical studies**, and we discussed the difference between interventional studies and observational studies. Clinical studies may estimate **incidence** and **prevalence** rates, risk factors, correlations, and temporal trends; the majority of studies, however, assess new diagnostic or therapeutic procedures, and take the form of interventional studies.

Aims of studies

In diagnostic studies, or diagnostic trials, two or more diagnostic procedures are carried for every participant. In many cases, a "gold standard" or reference method exists that is known to produce valid and reliable results, although it may be time consuming, expensive, or unpleasant for the patient. This reference method can be used to assess the correctness and **precision** of the diagnostic procedure under investigation. If there is no usable reference method, you can only measure the degree of correspondence between different methods, and you can wait for the subsequent course of the illness to confirm, or refute, the test results.

Diagnostic trials

In **therapeutic trials**, the success of treatment of a new therapy is compared with the success of a standard therapy in a comparable group of patients. In this context, randomized therapeutic trials play a particularly important role.

Therapeutic trials

There are studies that investigate the combined effect of diagnostic and therapeutic procedures, for example, the benefit of mammographies every 2 years for early cancer detection in women aged 40 and above. For that purpose, half of the participants are included in the prevention program—by **randomization** or as a cohort—and the other half are not. Every time a breast carcinoma is detected—be it at a prevention examination or at any other occasion—the patient is treated according to the state of the art. The benefit of regular mammographies is assessed in **terms** of disease and death rates, survival times, and measures for the quality of life.

Combined diagnostic – therapeutic studies

Of all study types, therapeutic trials are of the greatest practical use. This is why we discuss them in more detail. **Documentation** is a crucial task for therapeutic trials, as it is for all other types of studies.

Documentation in therapeutic trials

8.1 Therapeutic Trials

Objectives

Therapeutic trials are performed to test new therapies, especially new drugs, under controlled conditions. To prove its efficacy, the new therapy is compared to a placebo therapy; to prove its superiority, it is compared to the standard therapy. Moreover, in every trial the safety and possible side effects of the new therapy are assessed.

Methods

An extensive methodology has been established to develop and test new drugs. Complete and detailed documentation is necessary, in particular for studies that are submitted to the drug authorities for new drug approval. The study documentation is the basis of the authority's decision.

Phases

In animal experiments, the effects of a new substance are tested in respect of pharmacology, toxicology, and teratology (the potential of causing malformations in offsprings). Every single animal experiment is documented in detail. Human drug testing (clinical verification) always passes through four phases:

Phase I   Estimating the drug's side effects and assessing the pharmacokinetics and pharmacodynamics in a few healthy subjects.

Phase II   First testing of the substance in patients and within the designated field of indication, carried out with close supervision of the patient (test of efficacy and safety); determining adequate preparation (galenics), dosage, and regimen.

Phase III   Formal proof of effectiveness (where there is no convincing therapy yet for the target indication), or of superiority to the current standard therapy, under controlled clinical conditions.

– Approval of the new drug –

Phase IV   Application surveillance (therapeutic use studies) in a large number of patients in order to optimize the use of the new drug, and to assess its effectiveness, its safety, and its side effects under varying clinical conditions. These conditions include the application of the drug to patients who are commonly excluded from phase III trials, such as multimorbid or elderly patients.

There are documentary tasks in studies of all phases. These tasks are most demanding in clinical studies of phases III and IV, where you have a large number of patients in real and complex clinical situations; this is particularly true in studies conducted at more than one hospital or doctor's office. For those multicentered studies, it is particularly difficult to achieve the necessary **observational equivalence**.

Good Clinical Practice (GCP)

8.2

Description

Clinical studies that are submitted for the approval of a new drug have to meet a number of requirements, many of them concerning documentation processes. Together with the pharmaceutical industry and medical faculties, the drug regulation authorities have developed a set of guidelines for that purpose; one of them is called the **Good Clinical Practice** (GCP). There are other guidelines dealing with the manufacturing of drugs (Good Manufacturing Practice) and the performance of laboratory tests (Good Laboratory Practice).

The current version of the GCP guidelines was worked out by the International Conference on Harmonization of Technical Requirements for Registration of Pharmaceuticals for Human Use (ICH), founded by the U.S., Japan, and the European Union. A therapeutic trial that is carried out according to GCP today is acknowledged virtually all over the world.

The GCP guidelines, along with other recommendations on **clinical trials** (e.g., "General Considerations for Clinical Trials," "Clinical Safety **Data Management**," or "Structure and Content of Clinical Study Reports"), may be downloaded from ICH's official Web site at http://www.ifpma.org/ich1.html.

SOPs

One of the guiding ideas of GCP is to **document** a clinical study in a way that allows every single step to be reproduced afterward. To cope with the immense amount of documentation, **standard operating procedures** (SOPs) should be designed or adopted for every clinical study. The documentation of an individual study then has to refer only to the SOPs that were applied. Every activity, however, that was not carried out according to an SOP has to be described in detail.

With regard to documentation, there might be SOPs for:
- a patient's entry into the study and the randomized **allocation** of interventions,
- the management of **data**,
- the correction of data in case report forms,
- the closure of the study's database.

Extent and structure of the documentation itself is also guided in detail by these SOPs.

8.3 Study Protocol

Description

A clinical study today is planned carefully and in the fullest possible detail. All planning decisions are **recorded** in the study plan, or study protocol. The study protocol contains the design, or logical construction of the study—much like the building plan of a house or the blueprint of a machine.

The study protocol serves as a model for the **documentation protocol** described in section 6.2.

Elements

Important elements of every study protocol are shown in Table 8.1.

Persistence

The study protocol is, as you might say, the "constitution" of every study, and, as such, it is very hard to change. If changes during the study become necessary, formal amendments have to be passed and added to the study protocol.

Table 8.1 Important elements of the study protocol of a clinical study.

- Present state of knowledge and topic of the study
- Study objectives
- Design of the study
- Definition of the observational or experimental unit
- Inclusion and exclusion criteria of patient selection
- Definition of the treatment groups
- Definition of the target variable, or primary endpoint
- Secondary variables and confounders
- Procedures for patient inclusion into the study and group assignment (randomization, etc.)
- Examination procedures
- Masking of therapy groups (blinding)
- Treatment of withdrawals and dropouts
- Sample size, duration, and power of the study
- Principles of statistical analysis
- Collaborators and responsibilities
- Set of case report forms

8.4 Case Report Forms (CRFs)

Purpose

For data recording, every study needs a set of case report forms (CRFs) (sometimes called case record forms). They remind the physician or nurse entrusted with **data acquisition** of the data to be **captured**; they guide the examination process (e.g., "If rectal temperature >38.5°C, then take a blood sample for microbiologic analysis."); and they form the basic documentary evidence of the study.

Types of CRFs

The set of report forms of a clinical study varies greatly between studies. It may comprise only a few pages or take the form of a casebook to be filled in for every patient in the study.

These are important types of CRFs:
- Admission to the study (filled in once): This form is used to check whether a patient met the admission criteria, to determine the subpopulation (stratum) he or she belongs to, and to document the result of randomization.
- Initial examination (filled in once): Detailed state of health of the patient at the time of admission to the study.
- Daily, weekly, or monthly report (filled in regularly): Describes the course of treatment, including adverse events.
- Report forms for particular events, e.g., operations, infections, relapses, etc.: This form has to be filled in for each occurrence of such an event.
- End of active treatment (filled in once): Describes the target **variable** and the detailed state of health of the patient at the end of the treatment.
- Follow-up observations (filled in regularly at follow-up dates).
- Forms for observations made at other places, e.g., in pathology, at external laboratories, or at central study offices.
- Concluding form (filled in once): Describes the patient's state of health and the value of the target variable at the end of observation.

In the header of every CRF there is the (short) title of the study, the name of the form, the planned date of completion, the patient identification, and, for multicentered studies, the institution. The main part of the form, which encompasses the observed data, is finalized by the recording of the time of completion and the signature of the investigator. This makes each completed form a document in the legal sense, which has value as evidence.

Structure

Monitoring

8.5

To ensure high quality of the results, the principal investigator and the study management have to continually monitor the course of the study and the process of data acquisition. These are the most important monitoring tasks:
- Visit the investigating physicians in order to explain the study protocol, the SOPs, the case report forms, and the investigators' tasks; to assess the investigators' ability and willingness to collaborate and comply with the study protocol (prestudy visit).
- Continually monitor the number of patients admitted to the study by each investigator to evaluate the study's progress and to remove deficiencies in patient admission.

Tasks

- Regularly meet with the investigators to discuss all problems that arise during the treatment of patients. Experience shows that it is often documentation tasks that are unclear.
- Check all completed forms for **completeness** and plausibility; if necessary, compare the data in the forms with data in the **patient record** (source data verification).
- Deal with errors and queries that arise during data checks.
- Give concluding **information** to the investigators after finishing the study.

To perform these tasks, the principal investigator employs "study monitors." The monitors have in-depth knowledge of the study protocol, the SOPs, the CRFs, and all other formalities of the study. They visit the investigators regularly and check their data. Each visit of the monitor is recorded in a monitor's report, describing the study's progress, the questions raised, and the decisions made. In large multicentered studies, the work load for monitoring is substantial.

8.6 Auditing and Quality Assurance

Tasks

GCP requires the investigators not only to monitor the study process but also to prove the quality of the study's conduct, its data, and its results. To be able to give that proof, documentation must cover the entire process.

This task calls for the position of a quality officer, or auditor, a person who is, as far as possible, independent of the study monitors and the principal investigator. The quality officer monitors the monitors and reexamines a sample or all of the CRFs that have been completed and approved by the monitors.

Moreover, the quality monitor checks, or audits, all participating institutions (principal investigator, study office, central services in multicentered studies, study physicians and nurses, biometrical services, etc.). These audits check for adherence to GCP and to the study protocol; make sure that SOPs or local regulations exist and are met for every procedure; and evaluate the quality of the data and the documentation.

At the conclusion of the audits, the quality officer formally certifies the quality of the study's conduct, its documentation, and its results.

Processing of the Primary Data

Checking and Correcting Data

All data obtained in a clinical study are reviewed several times:

Checkpoints

- The investigating physician intellectually reflects on every statement he or she enters into the CRF.
- The monitors go through all completed forms and make inquiries about doubtful entries.
- Auditors check the CRFs approved by the monitors.
- As data are entered into a **computer** (see section 8.7.3), the software performs formal plausibility checks, e.g., as to whether the age of a patient lies within the boundaries set in the study protocol, or whether a 30-year-old woman is earmarked as "postmenopausal."
- Finally, the principal investigator or any other authorized person may review the data processed by the computer and make inquiries in cases of doubt.

For all missing data, illegible entries, and unclear statements, queries are posed in writing to the investigator who completed the CRF (data queries). As data are supplemented or corrected in resolution of data queries, they are always noted down on the original CRF. When changing a data item, the old value has to be crossed out in a way that it remains legible, and the new value be added along with the date of the correction and the signature of the corrector. If necessary, the reason for the addition or correction must be given on the CRF or on the data query.

In case of deficiencies

After correcting the CRF, the monitor or the auditor has to be informed, and if necessary, subsequent changes have to be made in computer-stored data.

Classification of Nonstandardized Entries

Nonstandardized entries are avoided in CRFs as far as possible, but have to be accepted in certain situations. Concomitant diseases, attendant medications, complications, adverse reactions, and general comments can often be provided as free text only. Free text does not directly yield to **statistical analysis**. Thus, for example, concomitant diseases are **classified** using the ICD-10, attendant medications using the ATC-**classification** and WHO's DDD Assignment (ATC stands for anatomic, therapeutic, chemical, and DDD for defined daily dose), and adverse reactions using the Adverse-Reaction Dictionary of the WHO. General comments and other free text for which no classification system exists have to be

When and how

supplemented with a simple yes/no classification: "Are there additional comments to this case?"

8.7.3   Secondary Data Acquisition

Data input

All data obtained and captured in a clinical study are analyzed with statistical software, and thus have to be fed into the computer. Investigating institutions that regularly take part in clinical studies increasingly use portable computers instead of paper forms to **enter data** directly into a screen mask. This portable device is either on line with the study database, or data are transferred through a daily or weekly remote connection.

Plausibility checks

During **data input**, the program performs comprehensive formal data checks. **Quantitative attribute** values must fall within the valid range, and qualitative values must be elements of the **value set**. There are tests for all conditional compulsory entries (e.g., the number of pregnancies is to be stated for all women over the age of 16) and invalid combinations (e.g., checkmarks for "retired" and "unemployed"). Missing values in the CRF are marked with a special symbol (e.g., a dot), in order to detect omissions in data input. A missing value for a compulsory **attribute**, as well as any implausible value, automatically leads to the printout of a data query to the originator of the CRF.

Second input and data comparison

Secondary data acquisition must be checked for misreadings from the CRF and for typing errors. Only small studies and those that are not intended for drug approval confine themselves to just one data input and subsequent proofreading. In all other studies, CRF data are fed into the computer twice, by two different persons. A computer program compares the first and the second input and marks all differences. An authorized person then tries to resolve the differences or otherwise generates data queries for the investigator.

8.7.4   Database Closure

Description

A large amount of medical data will never be absolutely complete or correct. Nevertheless, statistical analysis has to start at some point. The decision that no more values are added or corrections are made is a formal act and is called the closure of the database. The closure makes the data available for statistical analysis. Of course, the database closure is performed and recorded according to a special SOP. Moreover, the database is saved and safely deposited as a data file (sometimes even as a printout) at this moment.

Database closure constitutes a clear interface of responsibilities: the investigators and the monitors have to ensure the quality of the data; the study biometrician is to be held responsible for all errors in subsequent statistical analysis.

The entire stock of data has to be archived and kept ready for later analyses, for example, if an approved drug is suspected of causing adverse effects at some future time.

Analysis

8.8

Elements

The statistical or biometrical analysis of a clinical study, which is closely linked to the documentary tasks, typically is composed of the following elements:

- providing a basic descriptive analysis of all variables (or **attribute types**) in the database (for qualitative variables: relative and absolute frequencies; for quantitative variables: minimum, 1st quartile, median, 3rd quartile, maximum, mean, standard deviation);
- assessing data quality from a biometrician's point of view;
- deciding on the use of data of patients who could not be treated and/or observed according to the study protocol;
- characterizing the patients who had participated in the study;
- assessing the comparability of study groups;
- describing and assessing the effectiveness and/or superiority of the therapy under investigation;
- describing and assessing adverse effects, intolerabilities, and the safety of the treatment;
- performing an explorative analysis, i.e., to search for unexpected or conspicuous results in order to formulate hypotheses for future studies;
- assessing the **validity** of the study results.

Archiving the Trial Master File

8.9

Description

All documents and data that have been produced during a clinical study are collected in the trial master file. It consists of the investigator's brochure (containing everything that was known about the new drug substance and the new therapeutic procedure at the start of the study), the study protocol, the vote of the ethics committee, the randomization plan, the completed CRFs, the monitoring reports and data queries with all subsequent changes to the data, the protocol of the database closure, the protocol of the treatment disclosure in a study with masked treatment groups, the final database, the biometrical analysis report, the final study report, and all audit protocols and quality evaluations. The trial master file often requires considerable shelf space and has to be kept years after the drug has been taken from the market. To save space, the trial master file is often microfilmed.

8.10   Checklist: Data Management in Clinical Studies

Checklist

Clinical studies provide the scientifically convincing proof of effectiveness or superiority of a new therapy, the proof of therapeutic equivalence of (two) therapies, the assessment of the correctness and relevance of a diagnostic procedure, or the determination of prognostic criteria.

The demands on documentation are particularly high in clinical studies:

- A study protocol prescribes the course of the study in as much detail as possible.
- Data are recorded on specifically designed case report forms (CRFs), forming prolective documentation.
- Study monitors, who are independent of the investigating physicians, survey the study and check the CRFs. In addition, an external auditing, or quality control, may exist.
- Data queries are documented as well, along with all subsequent supplements and corrections.
- The are several standards guiding the design, the conduct, the analysis, and the reporting of clinical studies, especially drug regulation laws and the GCP guideline issued by the ICH (see section 8.2).
- According to these guidelines, each single activity in the study process must be reproducible on the basis of the documentation, and by complying to preset SOPs.
- In clinical studies, there is a need to classify, among others, concomitant diseases (using the ICD, for example), attendant medications (using the ATC classification and the DDD assignment for example), and adverse effects (using WHO's Adverse Reaction Dictionary, for example.).
- Data recording, data input, and quality control ("data cleansing") are concluded through the closure of the database. The clinical study itself ends with the biometrical analysis and the final study report.
- The extensive documentation of a clinical study is intended to guarantee the high quality of data, to make all study activities verifiable, and, in this way, to achieve worldwide acceptance of the results.

Exercise

8.11

More and more activities in clinical studies are supported by computers. What functions could an **application system** provide to support the documentary process in clinical studies?

Exercise 1

Concluding Remarks   9

In the preface we stated, "Careful **documentation** is essential in all fields of medicine and health care, whether it may serve the treatment of patients, compliance with legal obligations, reimbursement and cost analysis, **quality assurance**, or clinical research." Having read this book, you are now acquainted with the basic principles of **medical documentation** and in a position to participate in the design of clinical **data management systems** and use them effectively. But this book is only an introduction to the field. Some questions that were not addressed here will arise when you start dealing with a real system. Moreover, medical documentation is subject to incessant changes, due to new developments in health care and informatics, as well as to the ever-changing conditions of national health care systems. The suggested further **information** that we provide in the following chapter, which cannot claim **completeness** in any way, is meant as a guide to answer your pending questions. We would further recommend that you consult medical documentation experts.

Suggested Further Information   10

General References   10.1

There are many journals and other regular conference proceedings in medical/health informatics. We found that good places to look for current literature on medical documentation are the *Methods of Information in Medicine* (ISSN 0026-1270, http://www.methods-online.com), the *International Journal of Medical Informatics* (ISSN 1386-5056, http://www.elsevier.nl/locate/ijmedinf) and the *Journal of the American Medical Informatics Association* (JAMIA, ISSN 1067-5027, http://www.jamia.org/). The *IMIA Yearbook of Medical Informatics* (ISSN 0943-4747, http://www.med.uni-heidelberg.de/mi/yearbook/index.htm) provides a collection of selected articles from the most important health/medical informatics journals. You will find references to other journals if you follow the Web links given below.

important serial publications

We indicated a few Web links (URLs) in the text. As the Internet is too transient an environment to justify extensive link lists in a book, we confine ourselves to some starting points for your own investigations.

Web links

IMIA—http://www.imia.org
   Information portal of the International Medical Informatics Association (see section 10.4).
PubMed—http://www.ncbi.nlm.nih.gov/entrez/query.fcgi
   U.S. National Library of Medicine's free public access to biomedical literature databases, e.g., MEDLINE.
Health On the Net Foundation—http://www.hon.ch
   Access to quality-assured medical information and literature with a structured query interface.
Medical Matrix—http://www.medmatrix.org/
   An ordered and annotated directory of medical Web sites with a special section on computer applications and informatics; free registration.
Health Informatics World Wide—http://hiww.org/
   An extensive list of worldwide Web sites on health informatics, compiled by the University of Freiburg, Germany.

Standardization Bodies   10.2

The International Organization for Standardization (ISO)— http://www.iso.ch—is a worldwide, nongovernment federation of national standards bodies from some 140 countries, established in

ISO

1947. ISO's work results in international agreements that are published as international standards. These standards are adapted and refined by the national bodies for their country's purposes. For example, there are standards about terminology work (ISO 704, ISO 860, ISO 1087), the vocabulary of information technology (ISO 2382), and quality management (ISO 9000-9004).

For the field of health informatics, ISO has established a dedicated technical committee *ISO/TC 215* (see the ISO homepage, standards development, list of technical committees) which is organized in five working groups on health records and modeling coordination, messaging and communication, health concept representation, security, and health cards.

To find out about the national standards organizations cooperating with ISO, see the listing given at the ISO homepage, About ISO, ISO members.

CEN

The objective of the European Committee for standardization (CEN)—http://www.cenorm.be—is to promote voluntary technical harmonization in Europe in conjunction with worldwide bodies and its partners in Europe. CEN also maintains a technical committee on health informatics: http://www.centc251.org.

10.3   Education in Medical Documentation

Programs

In several countries, dedicated educational programs for medical documentation are offered, e.g., Health Information Administration / Health Information Technology (U.S.), Medical Record Officer (U.K.), Medisch Administrateur (The Netherlands), and Medizinischer Dokumentar / Dokumentationsassistent (Germany).

Moreover, every program in Health/Medical Informatics (H/MI) should comprise substantial courses in medical documentation. There are various programs in H/MI throughout the world. A number of universities offer dedicated H/MI curricula. Postgraduate and continuous education programs in H/MI are offered for health care professionals (physicians, nurses, health information administrators, etc.) and informatics graduates. For information on individual programs we refer to the directory of IMIA's institutional academic members at http://www.imia.org/inst_members .html and to IMIA Working Group 1 on Health and Medical Informatics Education at http://www.imia.org/wg1.

IMIA recommendations

Moreover, IMIA agreed on international recommendations in H/MI education, serving as a framework for national courses and programs as well as for the international exchange of students,

teachers, and courseware. For health information administrators, IMIA especially recommends knowledge and skills in the fields of
- information literacy
- health terminology
- coding systems
- the electronic health record
- evaluation methodology.

The IMIA recommendations on HI/MI education can be downloaded from http://www.imia.org/wg1/rec.htm.

Professional and Other Relevant Organizations   10.4

World Health Organization, WHO
     http://www.who.int/
World Medical Organization, WMA
     http://www.wma.net/
International Medical Informatics Association, IMIA
     http://www.imia.org/
Asia Pacific Association for Medical Informatics, APAMI
     http://www.apami.org/
European Federation for Medical Informatics, EFMI
     http://www.efmi.org/
Health Informatics in Africa, HELINA
     http://www.uku.fi/english/organizations/helina-l/
IMIA Federation for Latin America and the Caribbean, IMIA-LAC
     http://www.imia-lac.org/

For national organizations, refer to the list of IMIA's national member societies at http://www.imia.org/member_societies.html.

Information on Coding Systems   10.5

General

Côté RA, Rothwell DJ. The classification-nomenclature issues in medicine: a return to natural language. *Medical Informatics* 14, 1989: 25–41. ISSN 0307-7640.

Cimino JJ. Desiderata for medical vocabularies in the twenty-first century. *Methods of Information in Medicine* 37(4–5), 1998: 394–403. ISSN 0026-1270.

Ingenerf J, Giere W. Concept oriented standardization and statistics oriented classification: continuing the classification versus nomenclature controversy. *Methods of Information in Medicine* 37(4–5), 1998: 527–39. ISSN 0026-1270.

Rector AL. Thesauri and formal classifications: terminologies for people and machines. *Methods of Information in Medicine* 37(4–5), 1998: 501–9. ISSN 0026-1270.

Josef Ingenerf's Medical Terminology Resources,
http://www.medinf.mu-luebeck.de/~ingenerf/terminology/

ICD

World Health Organization, ICD-10 page,
http://www.who.int/whosis/icd10/
U.S. National Center for Health Statistics, Classifications page,
http://www.cdc.gov/nchs/icd9.htm
Fritz A, Percy C, Jack A, et al. (eds). *International Classification of Diseases for Oncology (ICD-O)*. WHO. Geneva: World Health Organization Publications, 2000.
U.S. CMS/HCFA's ICD-10-PCS Material page,
http://www.hcfa.gov/stats/icd10/icd10.htm

SNOMED

SNOMED site of the College of American Pathologists, CAP,
http://www.snomed.org/
Clinical Terminology Services (including SNOMED CT information) of the U.K. NHS Information Authority
http://www.nhsia.nhs.uk/terms/pages/default.asp
Côté RA, Rothwell DJ, Palotay JL, Beckett RS, Brochu L. The Systematized Nomenclature of Human and Veterinary Medicine – SNOMED International. College of American Pathologists, American Veterinary Medical Association, 1993.

TNM

TNM site of the International Union Against Cancer, UICC,
http://www.uicc.org/programmes/detection/tnm/
Sobin LH, Wittekind C (eds. for the UICC). TNM—Classification of Malignant Tumors. New York: John Wiley, 6th edition, 2002. ISBN 0-471-22288-7.

10.6   Basic Literature on Medical Documentation

Degoulet P, Fieschi M. Introduction to Clinical Informatics (Computers in Health Care). New York: Springer 1997. ISBN 0-387-94641-1.
Dick RS, Steen EB, Detmer DE (eds.). The Computer-Based Patient Record – An Essential Technology for Health Care. Institute of Medicine, National Academy Press: Washington, D.C., revised edition 1997. ISBN 0-309-05532-6. Text online at
http://www.nap.edu/books/0309055326/html/index.html
Donabedian A. The quality of care—How can it be assessed? *Journal of the American Medical Association* 260, 1988: 1743–8.
ISSN 0098-7484.
Feinstein AR. The problems of the "Problem Oriented Medical Record." *Annals of Internal Medicine* 78, 1973: 751–62. ISSN 0003-4819.
Feinstein AR. Scientific standards in epidemiologic studies of the menace of daily life. *Science* 242, 1988: 1257–63. ISSN 0036-8075.
Green SB, Byar DP. Using observational data from registries to compare treatments: the fallacy of omnimetrics. *Statistics in Medicine* 3, 1984: 361–70. ISSN 0277-6715.

Haux R. Knowledge-based decision support for diagnosis and therapy: on the multiple usability of patient data. *Methods of Information in Medicine* 28, 1989: 69–77. ISSN 0026-1270.

Haux R, Winter A, Ammenwerth E, Brigl B: *Strategic Information Management in Hospitals. An Introduction to Hospital Information Systems.* To appear.

IMIA Working Group 1, Health and Medical Informatics Education. Recommendations of the International Medical Informatics Association (IMIA) on education in health and medical informatics. *Methods of Information in Medicine* 39(3), 2000: 267–77. ISSN 0026-1270.

Leiner F, Haux R. Systematic planning of clinical documentation. *Methods of Information in Medicine* 35, 1996: 25–34. ISSN 0026-1270.

Rector AL. Clinical terminology: why is it so hard? *Methods of Information in Medicine* 38(4–5), 1999: 239–52. ISSN 0026-1270.

Rector AL, Nowlan WA, Kay S, Goble CA, Howkins TJ. A framework for modelling the electronic medical record. *Methods of Information in Medicine* 32, 1993: 109–19. ISSN 0026-1270.

Roger FH. The minimum basic data set for hospital statistics in the EEC. In: Lambert PM, Roger FH (eds.). *Hospital Statistics in Europe.* Amsterdam: North Holland, 1982: 83–112. ISBN 0-444-86383-4.

Shortliffe EH, Perreault LE, Wiederhold G, et al. (eds.). *Medical Informatics—Computer Applications in Health Care and Biomedicine.* New York: Springer, 2001. ISBN 0-387-98472-0.

vanBemmel JH, McCray A (eds. 1992-2000); Haux R, Kulikowski C (eds. from 2001). *IMIA Yearbook of Medical Informatics.* Stuttgart: Schattauer. ISSN 0943-4747.

van Bemmel JH, Musen MA (eds.). *Handbook of Medical Informatics.* New York: Springer 1997. ISBN 3-540-63351-0. Text online at http://www.mihandbook.stanford.edu/handbook/home.htm

Weed LL. *Medical Records, Medical Education, and Patient Care. The Problem-Oriented Record as a Basic Tool.* Cleveland, OH: Case Western Reserve University, 1969. ISBN 0-815-19188-X.

Thesaurus of Medical Documentation   11

Documentation Protocol of the Thesaurus   11.1

Documentation Goals

The terminology used in the area of medical documentation is not always clear: the same concepts are often defined and denoted differently. This ambiguity makes communication under certain circumstances very difficult and diverts attention from the actual discussion at hand.

To reduce this problem, we offer a clarifying contribution to the terminology used in medical documentation; for this we set four goals:
- select the most important concepts in the field;
- define each selected concept in such a way that it is clear and complete, but also short and comprehensible;
- give a preferred term for each concept;
- supply additional information to place the concept in the context of the field.

To meet these goals, we put together this thesaurus of medical documentation. This is not the last word on the terminology of medical documentation, but rather the groundwork for practical discussion.

Questions and Nature of the Task

We considered the questions that you, the reader, would turn to the thesaurus for. For example, your questions could be:
- What does term x mean? Or more specifically: What concept is represented by term x?
- Are there other terms for the same concept? And which of these should I use?
- Which other concepts are superordinate or subordinate to a certain concept?
- Does term y denote the same concept as term x? And if not, does it stand for a more comprehensive or less comprehensive concept? Or a completely different one?
- Where is term x used in the book? Where in the book is a certain concept dealt with independently of the terms that are used?

Design of the Thesaurus

To address the above goals and questions, our thesaurus contains all concepts needed to understand this book. For every concept, the following information is provided:
- the definition,
- a preferred term,
- alternative terms (synonyms),
- other concepts that are superordinate or subordinate to the concept or that overlap with it,
- reference to other concepts denoted by the same term (homonyms).

We offer the following possibilities to access the description of a concept:
- an alphabetical index of all terms,
- references in the text to words in the thesaurus (denoted in boldface),
- cross-reference to related terms and concepts within the thesaurus.

You can also use the thesaurus as a typical key word index by referring back to parts of the text where the terms are used.

Thesaurus Entries   11.2

Acquisition

data acquisition   **See**

Allocation

random allocation   **See**
Synonymous term: Zuteilung (German)   **Relations**
pp. 26, 72, 82, 83, 86, 111, 119

Analysis

data analysis   **See**

Anonymization

The removal of the person or patient reference (e.g., name, ad-   **Definition**
dress, and date of birth) from data objects.
However, remaining data may be sufficient to reestablish this reference, i.e., to reidentify the person (for example, when a patient
has an exceptional job and lives in a small community and those
details remain in the documentation). Reliable anonymization
takes precautions against reidentification and makes it practically
impossible.
Pseudonymization is a special form of anonymization. Here, patient reference data are replaced by a pseudonym (usually a unique
number, e.g., a surrogate key) and may be reestablished at any time
via assignment tables. Therefore, the organization responsible for
the safekeeping of the assignment tables of pseudonyms and patient identification data is subject to strict security demands.

Synonymous term: Anonymisierung (German)   **Relations**
Antonymous concept: identification
Specific concept: pseudonymization
p. 76

Antonymous concept

Definition

Two concepts are called antonyms if they both are specializations of a common generic concept while forming a pair of opposites regarding at least one aspect. Examples:
- *tachycardia – bradycardia* (with "abnormal heart rate" being the common generic concept)
- *fever – hypothermia* (but also: fever – normothermia).

Relations

Synonymous term: Antonym (German)
Integrative concept: concept relation
p.   18

Application system

Definition

A system of logical and physical tools assisting human users in processing information and knowledge.

The term is usually used for application software implemented on one or more computers (computer-based application system). However, the application system can include conventional tools and aids like phones, filing cabinets, paper forms, organizational plans, and procedural standards.

An application system has a memory of its own that permits the storage of data. The application system usually requires external information alongside it delivering information to the outside; thus, it often depends on the interchange of messages with other application systems.

Relations

Synonymous term: Anwendungssystem (German)
Specific concepts: computer-based application system, data management system

pp. 21, 65, 78, 103, 106, 108, 110, 111, 127

Attribute

Definition

Short for attribute type and attribute value. Examples of attributes are:
- brown hair (attribute of a person)
- admission diagnosis: suspected appendicitis (attribute of a patient's hospital stay)

The term attribute is occasionally used synonymously with attribute value or with attribute type.

Synonymous terms:	Merkmal (German), attribute value, attribute type (used in the corresponding sense)	**Relations**
Specific concept:	classifying attribute	
Partitive concepts:	attribute value, attribute type	

pp. 5, 6, 7, 8, 15, 16, 19, 20, 22, 25, 26, 27, 28, 32, 33, 36, 39, 66, 67, 68, 69, 70, 80, 82, 83, 84, 85, 91, 99, 113, 115, 116, 124

Attribute type

Category of attribute values used as a criterion for the establish-**Definition**
ment of a concept system (cf. ISO 1087). An attribute type may
take on the function of an attribute value with regard to a higher
level of abstraction. Example:
1st level of abstraction: attribute type: *gender*
                                values: *male, female*
2nd level of abstraction: attribute type: *patient's features*
                                values: *name, gender, age, diagnoses*
The term attribute is occasionally used synonymously with attribute type. In statistical analysis, attribute types are commonly called
variables.

Synonymous terms:	Merkmalsart (German), variable, attribute (used in the corresponding sense)	**Relations**
Integrative concept:	attribute	

pp. 15, 16, 17, 19, 20, 22, 25, 26, 28, 30, 113, 125

Attribute value

Value of an attribute type as observed for a particular object (e.g., **Definition**
the value *brown* of the attribute type *color of hair*). Attribute type
and attribute value form an attribute.
The term attribute is occasionally used synonymously with attribute value.

Synonymous terms:	Merkmalsausprägung (German), attribute (used in the corresponding sense)	**Relations**
Integrative concept:	attribute	

pp. 15, 16, 17, 19, 22, 30, 33, 84

Authorized term

Definition

Term of a documentary language. Authorized terms, or descriptors, are used to describe outside-world objects in a standardized documentation. Consequently, authorized terms are also used to formulate queries for data objects in a database.

The exclusive use of authorized terms in documentation reduces ambiguity and therefore is a measure of terminological control.

Relations

Synonymous terms:	Deskriptor (German), descriptor
Generic concept:	term
Intersecting concepts:	terminological control, preferred term

pp. 30, 31, 32, 35, 36, 37, 38, 89, 90

Axis

See Relations

semantic dimension

Synonymous term:	Achse (German)

pp. 34, 35, 37, 58, 59, 61

Basic data set documentation

Definition

Standardized documentation of a few particularly important attributes of all patients of a health care institution. The basic data set documentation permits the retrieval of all patients with particular attributes (e.g., specific diagnoses or therapies) and enables access to their health care documents. Moreover, statistics on those attributes can be produced and structured, for example, by age or gender. A health care institution thereby obtains a relevant current overview about its patients' characteristics.

In Europe, uniform attributes for outpatient and inpatient basic data set documentation have been suggested, and termed *minimum basic data sets* (MBDS).

Relations

Synonymous terms:	Basisdokumentation (German), clinical basic data set documentation (in this context)
Generic concepts:	clinical documentation, horizontal documentation
Partitive concept:	Minimum basic data set

pp. 27, 28, 63, 66, 67, 69, 109, 115

Bibliographic database system

reference documentation
Synonymous term: bibliographische Datenbank (German)
p. 110

See
Relations

Cancer register

medical register
Synonymous term: Krebsregister (German)
pp. 27, 69, 71

See
Relations

Capture

data capture

See

Casuistic analysis

patient-oriented analysis
Synonymous term: kasuistische Auswertung (German)
p. 105

See
Relations

Characteristics of a health care system

Mostly statistical data describing the characteristics of a country's or a region's health care system. These characteristics include the system's infrastructure (e.g., number of hospital beds available, number of neurosurgical departments) and performance (average length of hospital stay, mortality of a certain disease).

Definition

Synonymous term: Kenndaten des Gesundheitswesens (German)
Generic concept: information
p. 24

Relations

Class

classifying attribute

See

Synonymous term: Klasse (German)
Integrative concept: classification

Relations

pp. 16, 21, 24, 25, 26, 27, 28, 29, 30, 33, 34, 35, 37, 38, 40, 41, 44, 46, 52, 56, 58, 59, 77, 80, 85, 89, 90, 91

Classification

Definition

A coding system founded on the principle of arranging concepts into classes. A class sums up all neighboring concepts that are regarded as equivalent for the purpose of documentation. Classes are defined by the classifying attributes of their members.

The simplest classifications are categorical attribute types (see level of measurement) with few values (e.g., treatment success: yes/no; gender: male/female/unknown). More extensive classifications consist of a structured representation of their classes and the semantic relations between them (cf. ISO 5127/6). Classifications are often based on hierarchical concept systems.

A classification should cover the relevant domain completely (exhaustiveness), and the contents of any two classes should not overlap (mutual exclusiveness).

In documentation, the classes of a classification are often represented by means of a notation, or code (cf. ISO 5127/6). These codes make up the authorized terms, or descriptors, of a documentary language. The most important rule for applying this language, and basic principle of any classification: assign exactly one code (or class) to each object or fact.

Relations

Synonymous terms:	Klassifikation (German), classification system
Generic concepts:	documentary language, coding system
Specific concepts:	multiaxial classification, monoaxial classification
Intersecting concept:	classifying attribute
Partitive concept:	class

pp. 16, 20, 32, 33, 34, 35, 36, 37, 38, 39, 40, 41, 42, 43, 44, 46, 47, 48, 49, 51, 52, 57, 58, 59, 60, 61, 79, 80, 89, 90, 91, 123, 126

Classifying (assigning an object to a class)

Definition

Assigning an object to exactly one class of a classification. For the assignment, an object has to contain the classifying attribute of the respective class.

Because of the great variety of medical facts and the structural deficiencies of many classifications, the unambiguity or reproducibility of the assignment can often be reached only by means of explicit application rules (here: classification rules).

Classifying is often combined with coding.

Synonymous term:	klassieren (German)	**Relations**
Homonymous term:	classifying (constructing a classification)	
Intersecting concept:	coding	

pp. 23, 28, 30, 33, 34, 35, 38, 39, 40, 42, 45, 58, 72, 79, 85, 91, 115, 123, 126

Classifying (constructing a classification)

Constructing a classification. **Definition**

Synonymous term:	klassifizieren (German)	**Relations**
Homonymous term:	classifying (assigning an object to a class)	

pp. 23, 47

Classifying attribute

An attribute that defines membership of a concept in a certain **Definition**
class of a classification. The classifying attribute distinguishes the
objects in one class from the objects in all other classes.
In a hierarchical classification, the classifying attribute distinguishes classes only at a particular hierarchical level. For example,
at the disease level of a medical classification, the classifying attribute of all members of the class of infectious diseases is "etiology comprises infection." By this attribute they differ from congenital diseases or injuries.
On a lower level of a classification's hierarchy, the members of
one high-level class may be assigned to different sublevel classes
by another classifying attribute.
For example, the infectious diseases (classifying attribute on level
1) gastroenteritis, infectious hepatitis, and wound infection differ
in the location of the infection (classifying attribute on level 2).

Synonymous term:	klassenbildendes Merkmal (German)	**Relations**
Generic concept:	attribute	
Intersecting concepts:	class, classification	

pp. 33, 34, 40

Clinical documentation

Definition

Medical documentation whose objects are the observations, assessments, and plans that were made during the health care process of individual patients.

Frequent object classes of clinical documentation are case histories, examination results, diagnoses, therapies, and action plans.

Relations

Synonymous term: klinische Dokumentation (German)
Generic concept: medical documentation
Specific concepts: (clinical) basic data set documentation, clinical findings documentation

pp. 2, 3, 21, 23, 64, 103, 114, 116

Clinical findings documentation

Definition

Documentation of a patient's signs and symptoms, observed mainly during his or her illness. Examples: symptoms reported by the patient, results of physical examinations, laboratory results, x-ray results, ECG results, etc. In chronological order, this documentation is also called progress documentation. Standardization of the clinical findings documentation (see standardized documentation) can be done only for specific questions of interest as they arise, for example, in research or in quality management; it is usually restricted to limited study samples and attribute sets.

Relations

Synonymous term: Befunddokumentation (German)
Generic concept: clinical documentation
Intersecting concept: progress documentation

pp. 24, 67

Clinical register

See Relations

medical register
Synonymous term: klinisches Register (German)

pp. 71, 117

Clinical study

Definition

Clinical studies are performed to produce convincing evidence of the efficacy, superiority, or equivalence, as well as tolerability and safety, of a therapeutic procedure for a given indication (therapeutic studies) or to investigate the sensitivity and specificity of a diagnostic procedure and its benefit to patients (diagnostic studies).

In a broader sense, clinical studies comprise *observational studies*, where patient care is not to be influenced by the implementation of the study. Examples are case-control studies and cohort studies. In a narrow sense, clinical studies are *interventional studies*, where therapeutic or diagnostic interventions are varied systematically (e.g., by random allocation). Interventional studies are also called *clinical trials*.

A clinical study is conducted following a *study protocol* that determines all procedures of intervention, investigation, and documentation in order to ensure observational equivalence. The evaluation of clinical studies is a method of patient-group analysis and draws heavily on statistical methods (see statistical analysis).

Relations

Synonymous term:	klinische Studie (German)
Specific concepts:	clinical trial, therapeutic trial, diagnostic trial
Intersecting concepts:	patient-group analysis, good clinical practice (GCP)

pp. 7, 27, 63, 71, 72, 73, 75, 82, 83, 84, 85, 87, 93, 117, 118, 119, 120, 123, 124, 125, 126, 127

Clinical trial

clinical study

See

pp. 82, 84, 119

Code

A series of characters or numerals representing a concept or a combination of concepts and unambiguously depicting its position in a systematic context (of a concept system).

Definition

Codes are used as a simple and unambiguous way to label concepts and, at the same time, provide information about their position in a concept system.

Example: The ICD-10 code A74.0 labels an infectious disease (A), caused by chlamydiae (A74), in that case chlamydial conjunctivitis (A74.0).

Synonymous terms:	Notation (German), notation

Relations

pp. 1, 31, 32, 33, 35, 36, 37, 38, 40, 44, 45, 46, 47, 48, 49, 50, 51, 52, 53, 56, 58, 59, 60, 67, 107, 115

Coding

Definition

Assigning a code to an object and recording the code as a data object.

Relations

Synonymous term: notieren (German)
Intersecting concepts: indexing, classifying
pp. 1, 33, 35, 36, 38, 39, 51, 52, 58, 59

Coding system

Definition

A coding system is a documentary language based on a concept system. It defines and describes all authorized terms and arranges them according to the order of the concepts.
The authorized terms, or descriptors, of a coding system are usually codes that are used individually or in combinations to label (or code) objects in documentation (hence its name).
Typical coding systems are classifications and nomenclatures.

Relations

Synonymous term: Ordnungssystem (German)
Generic concept: documentary language
Specific concepts: classification, nomenclature
Intersecting concept: concept system
pp. 30, 31, 32, 33, 35, 38, 39, 41, 43, 47, 49, 50, 67, 81, 89, 90

Communication

Definition

Communication is the exchange of messages between persons or application systems.
Systematic communication, mostly an automated process between computer-based application systems, is an important tool for the establishment of logical data integration. Mutual understanding is a prerequisite for communication to work.
The set of physical and logical tools enabling communication between two application systems is called a communication link.

Relations

Synonymous term: Kommunikation (German)
Intersecting concepts: message, communication link
pp. 3, 4, 6, 8, 19, 22, 56, 77, 78, 104, 111

Communication link

communication		Relations
Synonymous term:	Kommunikationsverbindung (German)	

pp. 29, 69, 77, 108

Completeness (of attributes)

Completeness of documentation with regard to a certain data object: proportion of the data object's attribute types whose values were actually recorded (e.g., "Were all necessary data of patient Adams recorded?") If the answer is yes, completeness is given. Completeness is one of the prerequisites for observational equivalence. Completeness requirements also arise from clinical guidelines and legal demands.

Definition

Synonymous term:	Vollständigkeit (German)
Integrative concept:	standardized documentation
Homonymous term:	completeness (of data objects)
Intersecting concepts:	completeness (of data objects), observational equivalence

Relations

pp. 4, 8, 35, 37, 69, 71, 77, 80, 81, 113, 122

Completeness (of data objects)

Completeness of documentation with regard to a certain outside-world object class: proportion of the potentially recordable data objects that are actually stored in the documentation. Example: "Is there a data set/patient record for all treated patients?" If the answer is yes, completeness is given. Thus, completeness in this sense refers to the set of data objects, whereas the concept labeled by the homonymous term (see previous entry) refers to the set of attributes of a data object.
Many types of analyses require completeness of data objects.

Definition

Synonymous term:	Vollzähligkeit (German)
Homonymous term:	completeness (of attributes)
Intersecting concept:	completeness (of attributes)

Relations

pp. 4, 8, 66, 69, 80, 113, 129

Completeness rate

**See
Relations**

recall
Synonymous term: Rückrufrate (German)

Computer

**See
Relations**

computer system
Synonymous term: Rechner (German)

pp. 1, 2, 3, 8, 16, 21, 22, 28, 29, 30, 36, 52, 63, 65, 66, 77, 80, 85, 94, 103, 105, 106, 107, 109, 110, 123, 124, 127

Computer-based application system

**See
Relations**

application system
Synonymous term: rechnerbasiertes Anwendungssystem (German)

pp. 8, 108, 111, 114

Computer-based data management system

**See
Relations**

data management system
Synonymous term: rechnerbasiertes Dokumentationssystem (German)

pp. 1, 6, 29

Computer system

Definition

A digital data processing system. This includes stand-alone work-stations (personal computer, PC) as well as a central server con-nected to a number of clients or a complex communication net-work with several control units.

In the simplest case, a computer system is just a single computer (every computer is a computer system, but not every computer system is just a computer).

Relations

Synonymous term: Rechnersystem (German)
Specific concept: computer

pp. 29, 80, 103, 106, 111

Concept

Definition

Abstract unit of thought, based on the characteristics common to a set of objects. Concepts are not directly dependent on a certain language; they are influenced, however, by the social background of a language community (cf. ISO 1087). A concept is externally determined by its definition and labeled by terms or symbols.

A concept comprising a set of similar objects whose characteristics shall be documented in a data management system (e.g., the concepts "patient" and "hospital stay") is also called an object class (see Fig. 2.1).

Relations

Synonymous term: Begriff (German)
Specific concepts: object class, data object class
pp. 2, 4, 11, 15, 16, 17, 18, 19, 22, 23, 31, 32, 33, 34, 36, 41, 46, 53, 54, 55, 56,
     61, 82, 89, 90, 103

Concept relation

Definition

Relations between concepts may be hierarchical or nonhierarchical. Hierarchical relations are established by division of a superordinate concept into subordinate concepts. Hierarchical relations are either generic or partitive (ISO 1087).

In a *partitive relation*, the superordinate concept (the integrative concept) refers to an object as a whole and the subordinate concepts (the partitive concepts) to parts of it.

In a *generic relation*, the superordinate concept (the generic concept), comprises the meaning (the intension) of several subordinate concepts (the specific concepts).

Nonhierarchical relations may be *sequential* (e.g., predecessor–successor, cause–effect, process steps), or of any other, *pragmatic* type (e.g., similarity, periodic system of chemical elements).

Antonymous and intersecting concepts represent nonhierarchical concept relations.

The types of relations between its concepts determines the type of a concept system.

Relations

Synonymous term: Beziehung zwischen Begriffen (German)
Partitive concepts: generic concept, specific concept, inte-
                         grative concept, partitive concept, inter-
                         secting concept, antonymous concept
p.   18

Concept system

Definition

A structured set of concepts established according to the relations between them, each concept being determined by its position in the set (ISO 1087). The relations may be of the hierarchical, sequential, or pragmatic type (see concept relations).

A concept system is an essential part of each coding system.

By combining a concept system with a terminology and supplementing it with synonymous terms and other measures of terminological control, a thesaurus emerges.

Sometimes, especially in connection with knowledge-based systems, concept systems are called *ontologies*, implying that they provide a formal model of (a part of) reality.

Relations

Synonymous term:	Begriffsordnung (German)
Generic concept:	ontology
Specific concepts:	monohierarchical concept system, poly-hierarchical concept system
Intersecting concepts:	coding system, thesaurus

pp. 30, 32, 35, 41, 43, 116

Consistency

See Relations

referential integrity

Synonymous term:	Konsistenz (German)

pp. 90, 111

Content documentation

Definition

Data objects of content documentation (directly) represent objects of the relevant domain, e.g., patients, diseases, health care interventions. Content documentation provides a direct answer to the user's question, whereas reference documentation only gives clues to where the answer can be found.

Data management systems for content documentation are also called fact databases. Example: The database system *Chem-Bank* provides detailed information on potentially endangering chemicals. It is published by several federal authorities of the U.S.

Relations

Synonymous terms:	direkte Dokumentation (German), direct documentation
Antonymous concepts:	reference documentation, indirect documentation
Generic concept:	documentation

p. 63

Course of an illness

Chronological course of a patient's illness in interaction with the health care interventions carried out.
The progress documentation records the variation of one or more aspects of the course of an illness over time.

Definition

Synonymous term:	Krankheitsverlauf (German)
Intersecting concept:	progress documentation

Relations

p. 68

Data

(Singular: data item) A formalized, reinterpretable representation of information suitable for communication, interpretation, or processing (ISO 2382/1).
Formalization may take the form of discrete characters or of continuous signals (e.g., sound signals). To be reinterpretable, there have to be agreements on how data represent information.
Data are the input or outcome of an information processing step.

Definition

Synonymous term:	Daten (German)
Specific concept:	message
Intersecting concepts:	data object, document, information

Relations

pp. 2, 3, 4, 6, 7, 8, 9, 16, 19, 20, 21, 22, 23, 24, 25, 27, 29, 36, 52, 63, 66, 67, 68, 69, 71, 72, 74, 76, 77, 78, 79, 80, 81, 82, 84, 91, 94, 95, 103, 105, 106, 108, 109, 110, 111, 112, 113, 114, 116, 119, 120, 121, 122, 123, 124, 125, 126

Data acquisition

The first phase of data acquisition, or primary data acquisition, consists of *data recording*, in which the characteristics of an outside-world object are observed and secured, if necessary, in an original data record. The phase of secondary data acquisition, or *data entry*, follows, if necessary, to enter the primary data into the memory of a computer-based data management system.

Definition

Synonymous terms:	Aufzeichnung von Daten (German), data capture
Partitive concepts:	data entry, primary data acquisition, secondary data acquisition, data recording

Relations

pp. 3, 27, 29, 31, 69, 72, 79, 80, 81, 83, 94, 99, 100, 106, 113, 120, 121, 124

Data analysis

See

Relations

patient-oriented analysis, patient-group analysis, prolective analysis, statistical analysis
Synonymous term: Auswertung (German)
pp. 31, 52, 106

Data capture

See
Relations

data acquisition
Synonymous term: Datenerhebung (German)
pp. 7, 68, 79, 80, 81, 82, 84, 94, 120, 124

Data entry

See
Relations

data acquisition
Synonymous terms: Dateneingabe, Datenerfassung, Datenerhebung (German),
data input

pp. 29, 94, 124

Data input

See
Relations

data acquisition
Synonymous terms: Dateneingabe (German),
data entry

pp. 124, 126

Data integration

Definition

Condition of an information system in which each data item needs to be recorded, changed, deleted, or otherwise edited just once—even if it is used in several application systems. Data integration eases the burden of data acquisition and updating and it improves the documentation's consistency (see referential integrity).
Storing each data element only once is called physical integration. It eases database management and saves disk space. Logical integration is possible even if a certain piece of data is stored in more than one application system, with referential integrity being ensured by a systematic matching process. To achieve this, automated communication plays an important role.
Data integration is a prerequisite for the multiple use of data.

Synonymous term: Datenintegration (German)   **Relations**
Specific concepts: logical data integration, physical data
                      integration
Intersecting concept: multiple use of data
pp. 69, 77, 80, 110, 111

Data management system

An application system implementing documentation, or data man-   **Definition**
agement procedures. As with application systems we distinguish
between computer-based and conventional data management systems.
Coding systems, documents, repositories for data and documents, a
retrieval system, and organizational rules are components of data
management systems.

Synonymous term: Dokumentationssystem (German)   **Relations**
Generic concept: application system
Specific concepts: medical data management system, com-
                      puter-based data management system
pp. 4, 7, 9, 11, 13, 14, 16, 17, 21, 22, 23, 24, 25, 26, 27, 28, 29, 30, 31, 32, 39, 41,
     52, 73, 75, 76, 77, 80, 82, 84, 85, 86, 92, 93, 94, 95, 107, 109, 112, 119, 129

Data object

Set of stored attribute values describing an outside-world object.   **Definition**
The data object represents the object within a data management
system.
The structure of a data object, i.e., the attribute types and their
value sets, is described in a data object class (for explanation see
Fig. 2.1).

Synonymous terms: Datenobjekt (German),   **Relations**
                      (in databases:) data record
Generic concepts: data, object
pp. 8, 16, 17, 19, 20, 21, 23, 25, 26, 27, 28, 31, 36, 40, 78, 83, 84, 86, 94

Data object class

Definition

Object class for aggregating or abstracting similar data objects. Data object classes determine attribute types and their value sets, which set up the respective data objects that in turn serve to describe outside-world objects.

A data object class represents an outside-world object class within a data management system (for explanation see Fig. 2.1). Example: data object class discharge record—attribute types patient ID, discharge date, discharge diagnosis, etc.

Relations

Synonymous term: Datenobjekttyp (German)
Generic concept: object class
pp. 16, 17, 25

Data record

See Relations

data object
Synonymous term: Datensatz (German)
pp. 72

Data recording

See Relations

data acquisition
Synonymous term: Datenerfassung (German)
pp. 2, 4, 6, 8, 15, 16, 17, 25, 26, 27, 28, 29, 31, 32, 35, 36, 39, 67, 72, 76, 79, 83, 102, 104, 107, 109, 113, 120, 121, 122, 124, 126

Definition

Definition

A statement that describes a concept and allows its differentiation from other concepts (ISO 1087), using linguistic or other (e.g., formal) means.
pp. 1, 2, 6, 15, 17, 18, 19, 20, 22, 23, 36, 41, 44, 51, 52, 56, 59, 65, 79, 80, 81, 82, 83, 84, 85, 89, 94, 103, 104, 113

Demographic patient data

Definition

Data describing some basic characteristics of patients that are supposed to be relatively stable over the course of time (e.g., name, maiden name, date of birth, gender, address, etc.). These data are usually needed for identification and for administrative purposes. Demographic patient data are part of clinical documentation.

As demographic patient data are subject to change despite of their relative stability, they must be maintained systematically.

		Relations
Synonymous term:	Patienten-Stammdaten (German)	
Generic concept:	data	

pp. 76, 107

Descriptor

		See
authorized term		**Relations**
Synonymous term:	Deskriptor (German)	

pp. 36, 37, 38

Designation

label   **See**

Dimension

semantic dimension   **See**

Document

A (more or less) structured accumulation of data (usually paper-based or electronic), primarily intended for human perception. A document's data originate from an organizational context (e.g., an admission form is the record of an admission interview, a laboratory result sheet contains the results of one or more tests performed in the laboratory). A document can be exchanged as a unit between the users of a data management system and between application systems.

Definition

		Relations
Synonymous term:	Dokument (German)	
Intersecting concepts:	data, message, data object	

pp. 1, 2, 6, 13, 21, 22, 23, 28, 30, 33, 63, 64, 65, 66, 67, 68, 72, 77, 78, 107, 108, 109, 113, 114, 115, 119, 121, 125

Document carrier

Any medium for the physical expression of a document. Document carriers may be sheets of paper, x-ray films, file cards (or other

Definition

conventional media) as well as magnetic disks, chip cards, optical disks (or other electronic media).

Relations   Synonymous terms: Dokumententräger (German),
                                           storage medium

pp. 21, 23, 28, 65, 66, 113, 114

Documentary language

Definition   A formalized language used to describe objects (including documents) and facts with the goal of storing and retrieving (cf. ISO 5127/6). A documentary language consists of a set of authorized terms, or descriptors, which are used to form the descriptions according to a set of specific rules (the grammar of the documentary language).

High-level documentary languages take the form of coding systems or even thesauri in order to make them comprehensible and usable. Very simple documentary languages, however, can take the form of lists of descriptors or value sets.

The use of documentary languages is typical for standardized documentation.

Relations   Synonymous term: Dokumentationssprache (German)
                Specific concepts: coding system, classification, nomenclature
                Intersecting concept: concept system

pp. 30, 31, 32, 41

Documentation

Definition   The methods and activities of collecting, indexing, ordering, storing, and retrieving information in order to answer specific questions or to fulfill specific tasks.

Information is often contained in documents. To retrieve documents containing a certain piece of information, they previously must have been indexed accordingly.

Relations   Synonymous term: Dokumentation (German)
                Specific concepts: medical documentation, content documentation, reference documentation, horizontal documentation, vertical documentation, standardized documentation

pp. 1, 2, 3, 4, 5, 6, 7, 8, 9, 11, 12, 13, 15, 16, 19, 21, 25, 26, 27, 28, 30, 31, 33, 35, 36, 37, 41, 63, 64, 68, 69, 72, 73, 74, 75, 76, 77, 78, 79, 80, 81, 82, 83, 84, 85,

86, 87, 89, 90, 93, 94, 99, 102, 103, 104, 107, 114, 117, 118, 119, 122, 126, 129

Documentation protocol

The documentation protocol is the blueprint of a data management system, i.e., a detailed description of its planned elements and structure, deduced from given documentation objectives. Thus, it is a tool for the systematic planning of a data management system. The study protocol, which has become a standard for planning and conducting clinical trials, serves as a model for the documentation protocol. Figure 6.1 shows an example of the structure of a documentation protocol.

Definition

Synonymous term: Dokumentationsprotokoll (German)
Integrative concept: systematic planning of data management
                       systems

Relations

pp. 93, 95, 102, 116, 120

Electronic patient record

A complete or partial patient record stored on an electronic storage medium, or document carrier. Given this definition, every computer-based application system with clinical data management functionality contains at least a partial electronic patient record.

Synonymous term: elektronische Krankenakte (German)
Generic concept: patient record

Relations

pp. 63, 65, 73, 103, 109, 112, 113, 114, 115, 116

Entry

data entry

See

Epidemiological register

medical register
Synonymous term: epidemiologisches Register (German)
p. 71

See
Relations

Exactness

See Relations

reliability
Synonymous term: Genauigkeit (German)

Fact database

See Relations

content documentation
Synonymous term: Faktendatenbank (German)

Free documentation

See Relations

standardized documentation
Synonymous term: freie Dokumentation (German)

GCP

See

Good Clinical Practice

Generic concept

Definition

The superordinate concept of a generic concept relation in a hier-archical concept system. A generic concept comprises the meaning (the intension) of several subordinate concepts, called specific concepts. The frequently used term *generic term* is somewhat in-accurate, as it is not the term that is superordinate, but the concept it labels.
Example:
Generic concept *Lung diseases*—Specific concepts *Pneumonia, Pulmonary emphysema, Pneumonedema.*

Relations

Synonymous terms: Generalisierung (German),
    generic term (in the corresponding sense)
Antonymous concept: specific concept
Integrative concept: concept relation
p. 18

Good Clinical Practice (GCP)

Definition

Clinical trials put a strain on patients and are expensive. Results should be accepted widely and internationally. To achieve greater harmonization in the investigation and registration process of new

pharmaceuticals, the regulatory authorities of Europe, Japan, and the United States and experts from the pharmaceutical industry in the three regions joined in the International Conference on Harmonisation of Technical Requirements for Registration of Pharmaceuticals for Human Use (ICH) (see section 9.2.3).
The ICH developed guidelines for designing, conducting, recording, and reporting clinical trials. Some of these guidelines are called Good Clinical Practice. Compliance with this standard provides public assurance that the rights, safety, and well-being of trial subjects are protected, consistent with the principles of the Declaration of Helsinki, and that the clinical trial data are credible. Standard operation procedures (SOPs) play an important part in the implementation of GCP. The latest version of the GCP guidelines is published at ICH's Web site at http://www.ifpma.org/ich5.html.

Intersecting concept:	clinical trial	**Relations**
Partitive concept:	standard operating procedure (SOP)	

pp. 72, 119

Health care institution

An institution performing tasks in the field of immediate patient care. Examples are doctors' practices, hospitals, nursing homes, physiotherapeutic institutions, diagnostic advice centers, etc.
Patients come to health care institutions to receive health care interventions.

Definition

Synonymous term:	medizinische Versorgungseinrichtung (German)	**Relations**

pp. 4, 5, 6, 9, 24, 33, 39, 63, 64, 66, 67, 69, 70, 71, 73, 77, 78, 79, 81, 82, 84, 113, 116

Health care intervention

Action taken on a patient with the goal to prevent, diagnose, or treat a disease, or to rehabilitate the patient after an accident, surgery, or a disease. In general, health care interventions are carried out by health care professionals, working at a health care institution.

Definition

Synonymous term:	medizinische Versorgungsmaßnahme (German)	**Relations**

pp. 2, 4, 5, 27, 47, 70, 79, 83, 103

Hierarchical coding system

coding system
Synonymous term: hierarchisches Ordnungssystem (German)

p. 90

Hierarchical concept system

concept system
Synonymous term: hierarchisches Begriffssystem (German)
pp. 36, 90

Hit rate

precision
Synonymous term: Trefferrate (German)

Homonymous term

Definition

A term is said to be homonymous if it serves to label different concepts. Examples:
– ventricle for heart ventricle or for brain ventricle
– SLE for systemic lupus erythematosus or for St. Louis encephalitis.

In systematic documentation, all homonymous terms have to be clarified by making additions, like those we made to the "completeness" and "classifying" entries in this thesaurus.

Relations

Synonymous term: Homonym (German)
Antonymous concept: synonymous term
Generic concept: term
p.   18, 31

Horizontal documentation

Definition

Broad documentation providing few attributes of many data objects.

Relations

Synonymous term: horizontale Dokumentation (German)
Antonymous concept: vertical documentation
Generic concept: documentation

Specific concept: basic data set documentation
pp. 27, 30

Hospital information system

information system   **See**
Synonymous term: Krankenhausinformationssystem (Ger-   **Relations**
                         man)
pp. 63, 69, 73, 103, 104, 106, 107, 108, 109, 110, 111, 112

ICD, ICD-CM, ICD-O

International Classification of Diseases   **See**

ICPM

International Classification of Procedures in Medicine   **See**

Incidence, incidence rate

prevalence   **See**
Synonymous terms: Inzidenz, Inzidenzrate (German)   **Relations**
pp. 24, 71, 72, 117

Indexing

Labeling an object by assigning one or more authorized terms of a   **Definition**
nomenclature.
When labeling the contents of a document, its meaning (or message) has to be grasped before it can be indexed.
Indexing is often combined with coding.

Synonymous term: indexieren (German)   **Relations**
Intersecting concept: coding
pp. 36, 37, 38, 39, 40, 42, 52, 53, 73, 115

Indexing and retrieval language

nomenclature   **See**
Synonymous term: Indexierungs- und Retrievalsprache   **Relations**
                         (German)

Indirect documentation

See
Relations

reference documentation
Synonymous term: Verweisdokumentation (German)
p. 28

Information

Definition

Knowledge concerning objects, such as facts, events, things, processes, or ideas, including concepts, that within a certain context
have a particular meaning (ISO 2382/1).
Information in the narrow sense is the knowledge about concrete
objects (patients, laboratory results, and the like) in contrast to
knowledge about concepts (diseases, therapeutic methods, etc.)—
medical information in contrast to medical knowledge.

Relations

Specific concepts: characteristic data of health service,
                        medical information, medical knowledge
Intersecting concept: data
pp. 1, 2, 3, 4, 5, 6, 8, 9, 11, 12, 13, 14, 16, 19, 22, 23, 24, 27, 28, 29, 30, 32, 35,
   36, 40, 41, 51, 53, 59, 64, 68, 69, 70, 73, 75, 76, 77, 78, 79, 80, 81, 82, 84, 85,
   86, 87, 94, 103, 104, 105, 106, 107, 108, 109, 110, 111, 114, 115, 122, 129

Information and knowledge logistics

Definition

Effort to make available
- the right information and the right medical knowledge
- at the right time
- at the right place
- to the right persons
- in the right form
by means of systematic acquisition and processing of information,
or representation of knowledge, respectively.

Relations

Synonymous term: Informations- und Wissenslogistik (Ger-
                      man)

pp. 1, 8, 9, 103

Information system

Definition

A partial system of an enterprise (e.g., a hospital or any other
health care institution) consisting of *information procedures* and
all human and technical *agents* in their role as information processors. Information procedures can be understood as a set of formal

and informal activities and processes in which information is stored, processed, and exchanged.

		Relations
Synonymous term:	Informationssystem (German)	
Specific concepts:	hospital information system, medical office information system, clinical department information system	

pp. 28, 57, 69, 103, 104, 105, 107, 108, 116

Input

data input

See

Integrative concept

The superordinate concept of a partitive concept relation in a hierarchical concept system. An integrative concept refers to an object as a whole, while its subordinate concepts (the partitive concepts) refer only to parts of it.

Definition

Example:

Integrative concept *heart*—Partitive concepts *myocardium, pericardium, cardiac valves.*

		Relations
Synonymous term:	Integrativbegriff (German)	
Antonymous concept:	partitive concept	
Integrative concept:	concept relation	

International Classification of Diseases (ICD)

The International Statistical Classification of Diseases and Related Health Problems (ICD) is basically a monoaxial and monohierarchical classification. The ICD is issued by the World Health Organization (WHO). It is the only generally and internationally established classification of diseases. The English version of the tenth and, up to now, last revision (ICD-10) was published in 1989.

Definition

There are a number of additional or specialized classifications for special medical fields, e.g., for oncology (ICD-O), dentistry, dermatology, neurology, ophthalmology, rheumatology, and orthopedics.

Relations Synonymous terms: Internationale Klassifikation der Krank-
                                    heiten (German),
                                    ICD
               Generic concept: monoaxial classification
               Intersecting concepts: ICD-O (special classification for oncol-
                                    ogy), ICD-CM (clinical modification,
                                    USA)
               pp. 43, 44, 45, 46, 56, 57, 61, 123, 126

International Classification of Procedures in Medicine (ICPM)

Definition The International Classification of Procedures in Medicine is a classification of health care procedures, especially of medical operations. It was published in 1978 by the WHO.

Relations Synonymous terms: Internationale Klassifikation der Proze-
                                    duren in der Medizin (German),
                                    ICPM
               Generic concept: monoaxial classification
               pp. 47

Intersecting concept

Definition Two concepts are called intersecting if they share important characteristics but also differ in certain aspects.
Example:
Toxic hepatitis – liver cirrhosis.
Typically, intersecting concepts are specializations of a common generic concept. Thus, antonymous concepts are also intersecting concepts.

Relations Synonymous term: Begriffsüberschneidung (German)
               Integrative concept: concept relation
               Specific concept: antonymous concept
               p. 18

Label

Definition Since a concept is an unobservable mental phenomenon, it must be represented externally, using a label. Individual objects can also have labels, which are often called names.

A label can be a symbol (e.g., a pictogram or any combination of letters and numerals) or a linguistic expression in a particular language (cf. ISO 1087).
The representation of a concept using purely linguistic means is called a term.

Synonymous terms:	Bezeichnung (German), designation	**Relations**
Specific concept:	term	

pp. 17, 18, 22, 27, 31, 32, 52, 111

Level of measurement

The structure of the value set of an attribute determines the level – or scale – at which it can be measured. Basically, there are attributes at a quantitative and qualitative level. At the quantitative level, ratio scales and interval scales are distinguished. Ordinal scales and nominal scales are distinguished at the qualitative level: see Table 2.1.
The value set of an attribute at the qualitative level constitutes a classification. (A simple alternative like "complications: yes/no" is the smallest possible classification.) In statistical analyses, absolute and relative frequencies can be determined for this kind of attribute.

Definition

Synonymous term:	Skalvenniveau (German)	**Relations**
Intersecting concepts:	qualitative attribute, quantitative attribute	

pp. 20, 22, 26, 33, 68, 85, 91

List of descriptors

Simple, monoaxial nomenclature, providing only a list of authorized terms to index objects.

Definition

Synonymous term:	Deskriptorenliste (German)	**Relations**
Generic concept:	monoaxial nomenclature	

p. 37

Logical data integration

data integration		**See**
Synonymous term:	logische Datenintegration (German)	**Relations**

pp. 69, 78

Mandatory documentation

Definition

In many countries, there are extensive legal and institutional obligations for documentation.

Relations

Synonymous term: Dokumentationspflicht (German)

Medical data management system

Definition

Data management system realizing procedures of medical documentation.

Relations

Synonymous term:	medizinisches Dokumentationssystem (German)
Generic concept:	data management system
Specific concepts:	medical register

pp. 9, 30, 41, 82, 89, 94

Medical documentation

Definition

Documentation of medical information or of medical knowledge. Important fields are

– documentation of clinical and paraclinical observations (including measurements and images) and of clinical assessments (including plans), usually related to an individual patient or case,

– documentation of medical knowledge, e.g., about diseases, and

– documentation of health care literature.

Medical documentation is shared by all health care professionals, such as physicians, nurses, physiotherapists, etc. It is realized by data management systems.

Relations

Synonymous term:	medizinische Dokumentation (German)
Generic concept:	documentation
Specific concepts:	clinical documentation, nursing documentation, medical knowledge bases, health bibliographic database systems

pp. 1, 2, 3, 4, 5, 8, 9, 11, 15, 23, 24, 26, 41, 63, 70, 75, 92, 103, 106, 110, 112, 129

Medical knowledge

Information about the state of the art in the medical and health care domain at a given time, especially with regard to valid terminology, established or suspected relations, permitted interpretations of observations, and recommended methods and actions.

Definition

In contrast to medical information in the narrow sense, medical knowledge refers to concepts rather than to objects.

To emphasize nonmedical aspects of health care, medical knowledge is also called health knowledge.

Synonymous terms:	medizinisches Wissen (German), health knowledge	**Relations**
Generic concept:	information	

pp. 8, 19, 24, 28, 73, 103, 104, 110, 115

Medical register

A medical data management system with a main emphasis on scientific research in medicine. Medical registers are characterized by standardized documentation of patient data and by a defined study sample (i.e., explicit inclusion and exclusion criteria). They are built with a number of predefined analysis questions in mind but are also used for exploratory analysis, or data mining.

Definition

Medical registers are designed to answer questions repeatedly and periodically to demonstrate temporal trends. Therefore, unlike in clinical trials, the termination of a study is usually undefined. While ensuring long-term comparability, the questions and the data management system are continually adjusted to new scientific knowledge and changing fields of interest. Data of a medical register is not suitable to answer questions that require random allocation of procedures.

Medical registers usually apply horizontal documentation, i.e., they comprise few attributes of many patients. Typically, they use methods of patient-group analysis.

The study sample of *clinical registers* comprises only patients of one or a few health care institutions, whereas *epidemiological registers* strive to record data of all patients in a certain region (e.g., a state) completely. *Cancer registers* are typical examples for epidemiological registers.

The organization hosting a medical register is sometimes called a medical registry.

Relations	Synonymous term:	medizinisches Register (German)
	Generic concept:	medical data management system
	Specific concepts:	clinical register, epidemiological register, cancer register
	Intersecting concepts:	patient-group analysis, medical registry
	pp. 63, 67, 71, 72, 73, 82, 83, 84, 85, 87	

Medical registry

See	medical register

Medical Subject Headings (MeSH)

Definition	U.S. National Library of Medicine's nomenclature for coding medical journal articles.

Relations	Generic concept:	coding system, nomenclature
	Intersecting concept:	polyhierarchical concept system
	p. 60	

MEDLINE

See	reference documentation
	p. 110

MeSH

See	Medical Subject Headings

Message

Definition	A message consists of data that are put together for transmission and are considered an entity for this purpose.

Relations	Synonymous term:	Nachricht (German)
	Generic concept:	data
	Intersecting concepts:	document, communication
	pp. 20, 21, 22, 111	

Minimum Basic Data Set (MBDS)

basic data set documentation   **See**
p. 67

Monoaxial classification

multiaxial classification   **See**
Synonymous term: einachsige Klassifikation (German)   **Relations**
pp. 41, 48

Monoaxial nomenclature

multiaxial nomenclature   **See**
Synonymous term: einachsige Nomenklatur (German)   **Relations**
Specific concept: list of descriptors
p. 37

Monodimensional classification

multiaxial classification   **See**
Synonymous term: eindimensionale Klassifikation (German)   **Relations**

Monodimensional nomenclature

multiaxial nomenclature   **See**
Synonymous term: eindimensionale Nomenklatur (German)   **Relations**

Monohierarchical concept system

Hierarchical concept system in which each concept is subordinated   **Definition**
directly to not more than one superordinate concept. In contrast, in
a *polyhierarchical concept system*, each concept may have several
superordinate concepts.
Monohierarchical concept systems are easier to describe and to
handle than polyhierarchical concept systems but are often only a
poor image of reality. For an example of the application to classifications see section 2.4.3.1. The International Classification of
Diseases and the International Classification of Procedures in
Medicine are also based on monohierarchical concept systems.

Relations Synonymous term: monohierarchische Begriffsordnung
(German)

Generic concept: (hierarchical) concept system

Antonymous concept: polyhierarchical concept system

Multiaxial classification

Definition Multiaxial classifications consist of two or more independent partial classifications. The respective classifying attributes describe an object within different semantic dimensions. The object is classified separately for each partial classification. The partial classifications may themselves be structured hierarchically.

Example: A pneumonia developed during a hospital stay can be considered from the aspect (axis) of pathology (e.g., inflammation), the aspect of location (the lung), and from its cause (e.g., nosocomial). For a further example see section 2.4.3.1.

Relations Synonymous tems: mehrachsige Klassifikation (German),
multidimensional classification

Antonymous concept: monoaxial classification

Generic concept: classification

Specific concept: TNM system

pp. 34, 35, 37, 41, 49

Multiaxial nomenclature

Definition Multiaxial nomenclatures consist of two or more independent (but complementary) partial nomenclatures. The respective authorized terms describe an object within different semantic dimensions. The object is indexed separately for each partial nomenclature.

Example: see section 2.4.3.2.

Relations Synonymous terms: mehrachsige Nomenklatur (German),
multidimensional nomenclature

Antonymous concept: monoaxial nomenclature

Generic concept: nomenclature

Specific concept: Systematized Nomenclature of Medicine
(SNOMED)

pp. 37, 38, 53

Multidimensional classification

See multiaxial classification

Synonymous term:	mehrdimensionale Klassifikation (German)	**Relations**

pp. 34, 89

Multidimensional nomenclature

multiaxial nomenclature   **See**
Synonymous term: mehrdimensionale Nomenklatur (Ger-   **Relations**
                        man)

Multiple use of data

Data captured (see data acquisition) once are used for more than   **Definition**
one data management task. To achieve multiple usability, data
management systems have to be planned in a way that the quality
of all acquired data is sufficient for the whole range of tasks they
serve. Another prerequisite is data integration on the technical
level.

Synonymous term: multiple Verwendung von Daten (Ger-   **Relations**
                        man)
Intersecting concept: data integration
pp. 6, 81, 94, 110, 111, 114

Noise

precision   **See**
Synonymous term: Ballast (German)   **Relations**
Antonymous concept: precision
pp. 1, 4

Nomenclature

Systematic arrangement of terms allowed for a documentation task   **Definition**
(authorized terms). Thus, a nomenclature forms a concept system
and at the same time constitutes a documentary language. The
most important rule for applying this language: Each fact can be
described using any number of authorized terms.

Synonymous terms: Nomenklatur (German),   **Relations**
                        indexing and retrieval language

Generic concepts: documentary language, concept system
Specific concepts: multiaxial nomenclature, monoaxial nomenclature

pp. 32, 35, 36, 37, 38, 39, 40, 41, 42, 52, 53, 60, 89, 90

Nonstandardized documentation

See
Relations
standardized documentation
Synonymous term: nichtstandardisierte Dokumentation
(German)

p. 26

Notation

See
Relations
code
Synonymous term: code

pp. 30, 44, 49, 54

Nursing documentation

See
Relations
medical documentation
Synonymous term: Pflegedokumentation (German)

p. 2

Object

Definition
Any part of the perceptible or conceivable world (ISO 1087).
Thoughts, events, and real or postulated facts are also objects.
Several similar objects can be summarized into concepts or object
classes.

Relations
Synonymous term: Objekt (German)
Specific concepts: outside-world object, data object

pp. 15, 16, 17, 18, 19, 22, 26, 27, 28, 31, 33, 34, 35, 36, 37, 38, 40, 77, 86, 90, 94

Object class

See
Relations
concept
Synonymous term: Objekttyp (German)

pp. 15, 16, 94

Objectivity

reliability
Synonymous term: Objektivität (German)

See Relations

Observational equivalence

Observational equivalence within a group of patients requires the same time points, duration, and intensity of observations, the same procedures of investigation, the same conditions and equipment for measurements, and, if possible, even the same observer. Furthermore, standardized documentation is a prerequisite for observational equivalence. When several groups of patients are compared, observational equivalence is needed within and between all of these groups. Of course, it does not make sense to strive for observational equivalence of patients with completely different disease patterns.

Observational equivalence serves for the comparability of data objects, especially when performing patient-group analyses. When selecting the attributes to be recorded, care has to be taken that they are objectively observable in order to achieve observational equivalence (see reliability).

Definition

Synonymous term: Beobachtungsgleichheit (German)
Intersecting concepts: standardized documentation, completeness (of attributes)

pp. 79, 83, 84, 85, 87, 119

Relations

Outcome quality

quality of patient care
Synonymous term: Ergebnisqualität (German)
pp 69, 70

See Relations

Outside-world object

An object of the observed part of reality that is described coherently within documentation. Examples from clinical documentation: patient Adams; hospital stay from January, 7 to 14, 1999, in the PMC; the disease tuberculosis. Example from a bibliographic database: the journal article titled "The Fall of the Medical Record," published in the *Annals of Internal Medicine*, volume 110, 1989, pp. 482–4.

Definition

In data management systems, outside-world objects are represented by data objects (the same goes for this book: have a second look at the examples above).

Outside-world objects are usually (more or less instinctively) assigned to object classes (the patient Adams, the disease tuberculosis, etc.; for explanation see Fig. 2.1).

Relations

Synonymous term:	Objekt der äußeren Wirklichkeit (German)
Generic concept:	object
Intersecting concept:	data object

pp. 17, 19, 21

Partitive concept

Definition

The subordinate concept of a partitive concept relation in a hierarchical concept system. A partitive concept refers only to parts of the superordinate concept (the integrative concept).

Example:

Integrative concept *heart*—Partitive concepts *myocardium, pericardium, cardiac valves.*

Relations

Synonymous term:	Teilbegriff (German)
Antonymous concept:	integrative concept
Integrative concept:	concept relation

pp. 34, 54

Patient care

Definition

The coordinated application of health care interventions on patients, usually carried out by health care professionals at one or more health care institutions.

Relations

Synonymous term:	Patientenversorgung (German)

pp. 1, 2, 3, 5, 7, 9, 11, 13, 26, 64, 67, 69, 104, 106, 112, 114

Patient record

Definition

The patient record comprises all data and documents generated or received during the care of a patient at a health care institution. Document carriers may be conventional or electronic media.

In its still most common form, the patient record is paper-based, contains a growing proportion of computer printouts, and is supplemented by an extra envelope or folder for x-ray images (see electronic patient record).

The patient record comprises a number of partial documentations (case history documentation, clinical findings documentation, summaries, overviews, etc.) with different objectives and different characteristics.

Synonymous term:	Krankenakte (German)	**Relations**
Specific concept:	electronic patient record	

pp. 2, 4, 16, 22, 23, 28, 40, 63, 64, 65, 66, 67, 73, 106, 107, 108, 113, 114, 115, 116, 122

Patient-group analysis

Analysis of medical documentation focused on the determination **Definition** of aggregated characteristics of predefined groups of patients. Due to the predominant use of statistical methods, it is sometimes equated with statistical analysis. Methodical problems arise mainly in the recruitment of groups of patients with comparable disease and living conditions and in providing further comparability by equal health care and data acquisition (observational equivalence). When interpreting the results, further problems may arise, e.g., due to the lack of structural equivalence between interventional and control groups.

Synonymous term:	patientenübergreifende Auswertung (German)	**Relations**
Antonymous concepts:	casuistic analysis, patient-oriented analysis	
Intersecting concepts:	statistical analysis, clinical trial, medical register	

pp. 25, 30, 33, 35, 71, 80, 85

Patient-oriented analysis

Analysis of a medical documentation focused on information **Definition** about a single identified patient.

A patient-oriented analysis is often called 'casuistic analysis', implying that one medical 'case' is the object of scrutiny.

Methodical problems in patient-oriented analyses arise with regard to the correct identification of the patient, the adequate display of the course of signs and symptoms, and the clear and concise representation of information.

Relations

Synonymous terms: *Patientenbezogene Auswertung* (German), casuistic analysis

Antonymous concept: patient-group analysis

Generic concept: data analysis

pp. 25, 68, 75, 76, 77, 78, 87

Physical data integration

See
Relations

Data integration

Synonymous term: Physische Datenintegration (German)

Ploetzberg [pløts'bɛrg] Medical Center and Medical School (PMC)

Definition

A hypothetical medical school associated with a tertiary care hospital. Most of the examples in this book are located at the PMC. The PMC is fictitious, but similarities with real hospitals are certainly not coincidental.

Relations

Synonymous terms: Medizinische Hochschule Plötzberg (German), PMC

pp. 15, 22, 39

Polyhierarchical concept system

See
Relations

monohierarchical concept system

Synonymous term: polyhierarchische Begriffsordnung (German)

p. 60

Precision

Definition

When retrieving data objects in a data management system: Let us denote
– D, the set of all data objects stored in the system;
– R, the set of objects relevant to the given query;
– S, the set of selected data objects for this query (result set).
(For explanation of the sets see Fig. 5.1.)
Then precision = $|R \cap S| / |S|$, with $|X|$ denoting the number of elements of set X. Precision is defined as the proportion of data objects relevant to the query among the selected data objects. Precision is 100% when the result set contains only relevant objects.

The complement (1 – precision, the proportion of irrelevant objects in the result set) is sometimes called noise (see Fig. 5.1; cf. recall).

Synonymous terms:	Relevanzrate (German), relevance rate, hit rate	**Relations**
Antonymous concept:	noise	
Intersecting concept:	recall	

pp. 36, 52, 60, 86, 87, 117

Preferred term

synonymous term		**See**
Synonymous term:	Vorzugsbenennung (German)	**Relations**

pp. 32, 56

Prevalence

The prevalence (or prevalence rate) of a disease is the proportion of people suffering from it in a defined population at a certain date.

In contrast, the incidence (or incidence rate) of a disease is the proportion of a population that contracted it within a defined period of time (usually one year).

Both prevalence and incidence are always related to a certain disease (e.g., myocardial infarction) or to a class of diseases (e.g., coronary heart diseases).

Definition

Synonymous terms:	Prävalenz (German), prevalence rate	**Relations**
Intersecting concept:	incidence, incidence rate	

pp. 44, 71, 72, 117

Professional secrecy

Health professionals have the duty to maintain confidentiality about everything they learn about a patient during their professional activities. Note that professional secrecy must even be kept with respect to other health professionals who are not involved in the care of this patient. Only the patient is authorized to relieve health professionals of their obligation of professional secrecy. Laboratory assistants, administration employees, health information officers, health informaticians, etc. all share this obligation.

Definition

Relations   Synonymous term: ärztliche Schweigepflicht (German)
pp. 76, 77

Progress documentation

Definition   Recording the course of a patient's illness and of the care process. Progress documentation focuses on the presentation of chronological changes. Typical forms of presentation are progress notes, progress tables, and progress charts (e.g., the fever chart). Examples: During anaesthesia, blood pressure, heart rate, blood oxygenation, etc. is measured every minute and the course of each variable is displayed in a chart. During the hospital stay of a patient, daily progress notes are entered into the record stating the current signs and symptoms, how they are assessed by the physician, and what the next steps to be taken are.

Relations
Synonymous term: Verlaufsdokumentation (German)
Generic concept: clinical documentation
Intersecting concepts: clinical findings documentation, course of an illness

p. 68

Prolective analysis

Definition   Analysis of documentation where the study sample is defined before capturing even a part of the data ("preselection"). In a *retrolective analysis*, the study sample is defined after having captured at least part of the data ("postselection"). A prolective analysis allows data acquisition to be planned and aligned specifically to the posed questions, whereas in the case of retrolectivity, the investigator has to rely on data that were recorded without knowing the specific questions, and that often turn out to be insufficient to answer them.

Relations
Synonymous term: prolektive Auswertung (German)
Antonymous concept: retrolective analysis
Generic concept: data analysis
p. 68, 94

Prospective study

In a prospective study ("looking ahead") possible effects of an assumed cause are investigated. In contrast, a study looking for the possible cause to an effect already observed is called *retrospective*. Example: Observing smokers and nonsmokers (smoking as the assumed cause) over a certain period of time with regard to affections of the respiratory organs is a prospective investigation. Studies of this kind are called cohort studies because one or more cohorts of people are being observed.

Conversely, questioning patients with lung cancer about their smoking habits is a retrospective investigation. A study analyzing not only patients (cases) but healthy people as well (controls), and comparing the results, is termed a case-control study .

Definition

Synonymous term: prospektive Studie (German)
Antonymous concept: retrospective study
pp. 83, 94

Relations

Pseudonymization

anonymization
Synonymous term: Pseudonymisierung (German)

See Relations

Qualitative attribute

level of measurement
Synonymous term: qualitative Merkmalsart (German)
p. 20

See Relations

Quality assurance

quality management
Synonymous term: Qualitätssicherung (German)
p. 129

See Relations

Quality of the care process

quality of patient care
Synonymous term: Prozessqualität (German)
p. 69, 70

See Relations

Quality of a health care institution's structure

See Relations

quality of patient care
Synonymous term: Strukturqualität (German)

Quality indicator

See Relations

quality monitoring
Synonymous term: Qualitätsindikator (German)
pp. 36, 70, 73, 79, 81

Quality management

Definition

All activities of a health care institution's management to assure and continuously improve the quality of patient care. This includes setting the goals, defining the responsibilities, and establishing and monitoring the processes to realize these goals.

Relations

Synonymous term: Qualitätsmanagement (German)
Partitive concepts: quality assurance, quality monitoring
Intersecting concept: quality of patient care
pp. 5, 6, 9, 63, 69, 70, 76, 79, 80, 110

Quality monitoring

Definition

A planned and systematic observation of specific attributes (quality indicators) of a defined set of health care interventions that are chosen to be, in a way, representative of the whole care process.
As a subtask of quality management, quality monitoring serves to identify problems. A problem analysis usually follows. The success of any problem-solving activities can (and should) be checked again by quality monitoring.

Relations

Synonymous term: Qualitätsmonitoring (German)
Integrative concept: quality management
Partitive concept: quality indicator
pp. 5, 70, 79

Quality of patient care

Definition

Quality of patient care in the narrow sense is the degree to which patient care improves or stabilizes the health of a patient, measured by what could be expected by his or her initial condition (*out-come* quality). Outcome quality depends on the quality of the *structure* of the health care institution (Is there sufficient staff and are they well trained? Is the technical equipment adequate and operative?) and on the quality of the care *process* (Have all appropriate actions been taken and been well performed?).

There are no absolute measures for expected outcome, appropriate actions, sufficient staff, or adequate equipment—the assessment requires a health care system to establish specific criteria for good patient care under the given technical, financial, and political constraints.

Synonymous term:	Qualität der Patientenversorgung (German)	**Relations**
Partitive concepts:	quality of a health care institution's structure, quality of the care process, outcome quality	
Intersecting concept:	quality management	

pp. 2, 5, 43, 69, 73, 104, 110

Quantitative attribute

level of measurement		**See**
Synonymous term:	quantitative Merkmalsart (German)	**Relations**

pp. 78, 85, 124

Random allocation, randomization

To determine the effects of an intervention (typically a particular therapy or prophylaxis) with statistical methods, patients are assigned to the experimental group or to the control group strictly by chance. Random allocation is the best method to achieve (on average) structural equivalence of the groups concerning all known and unknown influences.

Definition

Synonymous terms:	Randomisierte Zuteilung, Randomisierung (German), randomization	**Relations**

pp. 84, 117, 121, 125

Recall

Definition

When retrieving data objects in a data management system: Let us denote
- *D*, the set of all data objects stored in the system;
- *R*, the set of objects relevant to the given query;
- *S*, the set of selected data objects for this query (result set).

Then recall = $|R \cap S| \, / \, |R|$, with $|X|$ denoting the number of elements of set *X*. Recall is defined as the proportion of relevant objects selected by the query. Recall is 100% when the result set contains all relevant objects. It is obvious that recall in reality can rarely be determined since the number of relevant but not selected objects is generally unknown (see Fig. 5.1, cf. precision).

Relations

Synonymous terms:	Vollzähligkeitsrate (German), completeness rate
Intersecting concept:	precision

pp. 36, 52, 60, 86, 87

Recording

See

data recording

Reference documentation

Definition

The data objects of reference documentation represent objects that are, in turn, data objects of another data management system, e.g., journal articles and monographs in a library or patient records in a hospital's archives. Therefore, a successful query does not provide the user with the information or knowledge he or she seeks directly, but with a reference to its presumed storage location. A typical example for reference documentation is a bibliographic database system (containing no full text articles or books).

An important online bibliographic database system in the field of medicine is MEDLINE, published by the U.S. National Library of Medicine.

Relations

Synonymous terms:	indirekte Dokumentation (German), indirect documentation
Antonymous concept:	content documentation
Generic concept:	documentation
Specific concept:	bibliographic database system

pp. 28, 64

Referential integrity

A characteristic of distributed databases, indicating the consistency of all stored data. In the context of clinical documentation this means, for example, that data of one patient stored in different databases and application systems can be assigned to that patient unambiguously and contain no contradictions in themselves (e.g., different spellings of the patient's name, or different times for the start of a treatment).
Possible inconsistencies have to be identified and solved regularly, e.g., by systematic communication.
Referential integrity is an important prerequisite for logical data integration. Data complying with referential integrity are called consistent.

Definition

Synonymous terms:	referentielle Integrität (German), consistency

Relations

pp. 76, 78, 111

Reliability

When describing an object by assigning an attribute value or an authorized term: degree of agreement when an object is described repeatedly
- at different points in time (reproducibility aspect)
- by different persons (objectivity aspect).

Definition

Synonymous term:	Reproduzierbarkeit (German)
Partitive concepts:	objectivity, reproducibility
Intersecting concept:	validity

Relations

pp. 6, 27, 58, 80, 84, 92

Representativity

Characteristic of a study sample to agree in the distribution of all possible confounding factors with the target population.
Representativity is necessary in order to generalize the observed results from the study sample to the target population. To reach representativity, certain sampling procedures have to be applied (random sampling, stratification, micro-census). Clinical documentation often has to do without these methods; in these cases, the target population can be constructed as a cautious generaliza-

Definition

tion of the study sample—basically the future patients of the documenting institution or of a comparable institution.

Relations Synonymous term: Repräsentativität (German)
pp. 85

Reproducibility

See   reliability
Relations Synonymous term: Reproduzierbarkeit (German)

Retrolective analysis

See   prolective analysis
Relations Synonymous term: retrolektive Auswertung (German)
p. 94

Retrospective study

See   prospective study
Relations Synonymous term: retrospektive Studie (German)
p. 83

Semantic dimension

Definition Viewpoint, or aspect, along which the structure of a concept system is arranged. A concept system can be based on several semantic dimensions.
Examples:
- In a system of disease concepts, typical semantic dimensions are etiology, topography, morphology, pathophysiology.
- In a taxonomy of pain sensations, one can think of dimensions like type, intensity, chronology, localization, or trigger events.

Relations Synonymous terms: semantisches Bezugssystem (German), (semantic) axis
pp. 34, 35, 37, 38, 44, 53, 55, 58, 61, 89

SNOMED

See   Systematized Nomenclature of Medicine

SOP

Standard operating procedure

See

Specific concept

The subordinate concept of a generic concept relation in a hierarchical concept system. A specific concept comprises only a part of the meaning (the intension) of its superordinate term, called generic concept.
Example:
Generic concept *Lung diseases*—Specific concepts *Pneumonia, Pulmonary emphysema, Pneumonedema.*

Definition

Synonymous term:	Spezialisierung (German)	**Relations**
Antonymous concept:	generic concept	
Integrative concept:	concept relation	

p. 18

Standard operating procedure (SOP)

To assess the results of a clinical trial it is important to know how the trial was carried out in detail. For that reason, standardized work instructions for all important activities in a clinical trial—so-called standard operating procedures (SOPs)—have been developed in the framework of Good Clinical Practice. There are, for example, SOPs for patient admission, randomization, labeling, handing over, storing and returning the trial's medication, data control, data query and data correction, data release, etc. All tasks of a clinical study that are not guided by an SOP have to be described in full detail. Thus, SOPs reduce the documentation needs of a study. Furthermore, SOPs help in quality assurance and are developed by the enterprise initiating (paying) or carrying out the trial.

Definition

Synonymous term:	SOP	**Relations**
Integrative concept:	Good Clinical Practice (GCP)	

pp. 72, 119

Standardized documentation

Definition

Standardized documentation requires the uniform acquisition (see data acquisition) of certain attributes belonging to certain objects. For that it must be defined (1) for which objects, (2) which attribute types, (3) with which possible values have to be documented.
A documentary language is typically used for standardized documentation.

Relations

Synonymous term:	standardisierte Dokumentation (German)
Antonymous concept:	nonstandardized documentation, free documentation
Generic concept:	documentation
Partitive concept:	completeness
Intersecting concept:	observational equivalence

pp. 7, 26, 66, 71, 72, 77, 79, 81, 83, 84, 87, 116

Statistical analysis

Definition

Analysis of a set of data objects using statistical methods. The objective is to describe and compare one or more groups of outside-world objects (e.g., patients, cases). The most important measures of descriptive statistics are relative frequencies, mean, median, other quantiles, and measures of variability.

Relations

Synonymous term:	statistische Auswertung (German)
Intersecting concept:	patient-group analysis

pp. 9, 20, 72, 123, 124, 125

Storage medium

See Relations

document carrier
Synonymous term:	Speichermedium (German)

pp. 8, 114

Structural equivalence

Definition

Between groups of patients whose outcome is to be compared in a study: equal distribution at the beginning of the study of all patient characteristics possibly influencing this outcome, with the exception of the grouping criterion.

Structural equivalence (e.g., with regard to age, gender, severity of disease) is necessary to be able to attribute differences in the outcome to being the member of a certain group.

Structural equivalence with regard to all influence factors is achieved best by randomization. For known influence factors, procedures like matching or stratification can be applied additionally or as an alternative to randomization.

		Relations
Synonymous term:	Strukturgleichheit (German)	

pp. 83, 84, 85, 87

Study sample

The set of outside-world objects – represented by data objects – forming the units of observation in an analysis of the data management system. For certain analyses, the study sample may be limited to a subset of all data objects by defining inclusion or exclusion criteria. Example: All patients treated in the internal medicine department of the PMC during the last 5 years. In a clinical study, the study sample consists of all patients enrolled in the study.

Definition

A study sample must be representative of the target population; otherwise the results cannot be generalized. Sometimes, there is no need to generalize and the results of the analysis only pertain to the study sample itself (e.g., in an analysis of the catchment area of the internal medicine department of the PMC in the last 5 years).

		Relations
Synonymous term:	Untersuchungskollektiv (German)	
Intersecting concept:	target population	

pp. 6, 68, 71, 82, 83, 84, 94

Surrogate key

An unambiguous, automatically assigned, and unchangeable key attribute for the identification of a data object. Example: serial numbers, uniquely assigned to all patients of the PMC.

Definition

The surrogate key avoids problems possibly arising with identifications bearing semantics (poor data entry, timewise variability, etc.). In some clinical data management systems, patient identifiers are calculated from a patient's name (at the time of birth), birth date, and gender; this is an example of an identification-bearing semantic.

		Relations
Synonymous term:	Surrogatschlüssel (German)	

pp. 76, 78, 111

Synonymous term

Definition

Synonymous terms are different linguistic labels for one concept. Examples:

- *car—automobile*
- *whooping cough—pertussis*
- *subacute spongiform encephalopathy—Jakob-Creutzfeld disease*

As a measure of terminological control, one of all synonymous terms for a concept is distinguished as the *preferred term*. In standardized documentation, the authorized terms of a documentary language are usually confined to only the preferred terms.

Relations

Synonymous term:	Synonym (German)
Antonymous concept:	homonymous term
Generic concept:	term
Intersecting concept:	preferred term

pp. 18, 31, 32, 36, 56

Systematic planning of data management systems

Definition

A way of planning data management systems by applying a given scheme for deriving the minimum system requirements from detailed objectives and side conditions. Systematic planning results in a documentation protocol.
Systematic planning of data management systems strives for methodological adequacy and efficient operation of the data management system.

Relations

Synonymous term:	systematische Dokumentationsplanung (German)
Partitive concept:	documentation protocol

pp. 92, 93, 95, 116

Systematized Nomenclature of Medicine (SNOMED)

Definition

The Systematized Nomenclature of Human and Veterinary Medicine (SNOMED) is a universal multiaxial nomenclature for the indexing of health care facts, including signs and symptoms, diagnoses, and procedures. SNOMED has been developed and has been continuously expanded by the American College of American Pathologists (CAP), starting in 1965.

In May 2000, CAP presented SNOMED Reference Terminology (SNOMED RT) as its most recent development. Currently, CAP joins efforts with the U.K. National Health Service (NHS) to combine SNOMED RT with NHS's Clinical Terms to form a comprehensive medical terminology, called "SNOMED Clinical Terms" (SNOMED CT).

		Relations
Synonymous terms:	Systematisierte Nomenklatur der Medizin (German), SNOMED	
Specific concepts:	SNOMED RT, SNOMED CT	

pp. 52, 53, 55, 56, 57, 61

Target population

The set of objects or persons (here usually patients) to which the results of the statistical analysis of a clinical study or of a data management system apply. For a given target population, the study sample has to be selected representatively. For a given study sample, the target population can be constructed as a stepwise and cautious generalization of the study sample.

Example: A study sample of all patients of a doctor's practice in 1998 with the diagnosis diabetes mellitus type II is being observed. These observations may form the basis for inferences to the target population of all diabetes type II patients of comparable practices in the same region for the next 5 years.

Definition

		Relations
Synonymous term:	Zielgrundgesamtheit (German)	
Intersecting concept:	study sample	

pp. 83, 84, 85

Technical vocabulary

terminology
Synonymous term: Fachwortschatz (German)

See Relations

Term

label
Synonymous term: Benennung (German)

See Relations

pp. 1, 3, 7, 11, 15, 16, 17, 18, 22, 26, 27, 30, 31, 32, 46, 51, 52, 53, 56, 117

Terminological control

See
Relations

terminology
Synonymous term: terminologische Kontrolle (German)
p. 90

Terminology

Definition

An organized set of terms in a specific subject field, together with the definitions of the concepts they denote (or label) (cf. ISO 5127/1).
Terminological knowledge thus refers to the knowledge of a field's concepts, their meaning, and their labels.
Terminological control includes all measures of a data management system to define and differentiate concepts as well as to unambiguously assign authorized terms to them.
A thesaurus emerges by combining a terminology with a concept system and supplementing it with synonymous terms and other measures of terminological control.

Relations

Synonymous terms: Terminologie (German),
technical vocabulary
Intersecting concepts: terminological control, thesaurus
pp. 15, 17, 18, 19, 26, 53, 56

Therapeutic trial

See
Relations

clinical study
Synonymous term: klinische Therapiestudie (German)
pp. 82, 117, 118, 119

Thesaurus

Definition

Combination of a concept system and a terminology in a certain field of documentation, augmented by additional terminological information like synonymous and quasi-synonymous terms, as well as the degree of terminological correspondence between neighboring concepts (their semantic neighborhood) etc.
Thus, a thesaurus is a means of conveying terminological knowledge (see terminology) in a specific subject field. (We hope this is what our thesaurus does in the field of medical documentation.)
On the other hand, the formal representation of a thesaurus can, to

a certain degree, make the terminological knowledge accessible to computer-based application systems (making them knowledge based).

Intersecting concepts: concept system, terminology   **Relations**
pp. 11, 32, 36, 41, 60

TNM System

The TNM system (T = tumor, N = nodule, M = metastasis) serves   **Definition**
for the uniform description of the anatomical extension of malignant tumor diseases. It supplements topographical and histological descriptions of tumors coded, e.g., with the ICD-O, the supplementary oncological classification to the ICD.
The TNM system is a three-axial classification with some additions. For each tumor localization (mammary cancer, colon carcinoma, etc.) there are specific classes in the T- and N-axis.

Generic concept: multiaxial classification   **Relations**
pp. 57, 58, 59, 69

Unified Medical Language System (UMLS)

U.S. National Library of Medicine's meta-coding system to link   **Definition**
clinical cases to pertinent medical literature.

Generic concept: coding system   **Relations**
Intersecting concept: thesaurus
p. 60

Validity

In the analysis of a data management system, validity is the apti-   **Definition**
tude of an attribute to convey the characteristic of an outside-world object that is relevant for the analysis. Example: The attribute "total cholesterol $\geq$240 mg/dL" is only of limited validity for the characteristic of a patient to be at risk of a heart attack. (In the end, for a patient only those attributes are relevant that affect the quality or duration of his or her life.)
The empirical examination of an attribute's validity requires a reliable external criterion (in the example above this could be the heart attack rate of patients with increased total cholesterol over 10 years.)

Relations

Synonymous term: Validität (German)
Intersecting concept: reliability
pp. 59, 84, 113, 125

Value range

See value set

Relations Synonymous term: Wertebereich (German)
p. 91

Value set

Definition Set of attribute values that are allowed for a certain attribute type. For a quantitative attribute (see level of measurement), the value set can be presented in form of a value range. Examples:
– attribute type gender, value set {female, male, unknown}
– attribute type height in cm, value range [0;300]

A value set is the simplest documentary language (strictly speaking, a monoaxial classification).

Relations Synonymous term: Wertemenge (German)
Generic concept: documentary language
Specific concept: value range
pp. 15, 16, 17, 19, 20, 23, 25, 26, 80, 84, 116, 124

Variable

See attribute type
pp. 82, 121, 125

Vertical documentation

Definition Deep documentation providing many attributes of few data objects.
In patient care, this means the collection of many and detailed attributes of selected patients in order to answer a specific question. The study sample of a vertical documentation is typically chosen by diagnosis (e.g., all patients with rectum cancer), by therapy (e.g., all patients with pancreas surgery), or by diagnostic test (e.g., all patients with heart catheter examination).

Vertical documentation is mostly established in highly specialized areas of a health care institution or within the framework of clinical trials.

Synonymous term:	vertikale Dokumentation (German)	**Relations**
Antonymous concept:	horizontal documentation	

pp. 27, 68

Index   12

Page numbers in italics refer to pages in the Thesaurus.

Health Informatics Series
(formerly Computers in Health Care)

Behavioral Healthcare Informatics
N.A. Dewan, N.M. Lorenzi, R.T. Riley, and S.R. Bhattacharya

Patient Care Information Systems
Successful Design and Implementation
E.L. Drazen, J.B. Metzger, J.L. Ritter, and M.K. Schneider

Introduction to Nursing Informatics, Second Edition
K.J. Hannah, M.J. Ball, and M.J.A. Edwards

Behavioral Healthcare Informatics
N.A. Dewan, N.M. Lorenzi, R.T. Riley, and S.R. Bhattacharya

Information Technology for the Practicing Physician
J.M. Kiel

Computerizing Large Integrated Health Networks
The VA Success
R.M. Kolodner

Medical Data Management
A Practical Guide
F. Leiner, W. Gaus, R. Haux, and P. Knaup-Gregori

Organizational Aspects of Health Informatics
Managing Technological Change
N.M. Lorenzi and R.T. Riley

Transforming Health Care Through Information
Case Studies
N.M. Lorenzi, R.T. Riley, M.J. Ball, and J.V. Douglas

Trauma Informatics
K.I. Maull and J.S. Augenstein

Public Health Informatics and Information Systems
P.W. O' Carroll, W.A. Yasuoff, M.E. Ward, L.H. Ripp,
and E.L. Martin

Advancing Federal Sector Health Care
A Model for Technology Transfer
P. Ramsaroop, M.J. Ball, D. Beaulieu and J.V. Douglas

Medical Informatics
Computer Applications in Health Care and Biomedicine, Second Edition
E.H. Shortliffe and L.E. Perreault

Filmless Radiology
E.L. Siegel and R.M. Kolodner

Cancer Informatics
Essential Technologies for Clinical Trials
J.S. Silva, M.J. Ball, C.G. Chute, J.V. Douglas, C.P. Langlotz, J.C. Niland, and W.L. Scherlis

Knowledge Coupling
New Premises and New Tools for Medical Care and Education
L.L. Weed